ELEMENTS *and* METHODS *of*
HATHA YOGA
CLASS DESIGN

Including a template for assembly
and graduated methods of usage - For all
teaching styles and discipline levels

DAVID TRIMBOLI RYT

Disclaimer

Please note that I am not medically trained, therefore this text is not associated with the study or practice of medicine. This book implies many variations on current practice; any concerns regarding these should first be cleared through an appropriate healthcare provider or medically trained yoga practitioner prior to application.

I would urge anyone taking up the study or practice of yoga to consult with their physician first. It is important for yoga students to understand their limitations and practice accordingly. Also, consult a physician if during or after practice <u>any</u> concerns arise. Since yoga is a very internal practice, this pertains to emotional and psychological issues as well.

ISBN: 1-4392-6928-9
ISBN-13: 9781439269282

You can find further information on this text and supplemental resources at www.yogaclassdesign.com

This book is dedicated to

Veronica Zador,

shala teacher, mentor, friend.

Contents

0.0 Introduction

This book was written from a unique perspective, therefore I recommend that you read the introduction over thoroughly. This will give you the proper orientation and will greatly help in your understanding of this text.

0.1 Why I Wrote This Book

I have been an engineer since 1986. While I enjoy my work, it (as well as life in general) can be stressful at times. Throughout my life, I tried different types of exercise to alleviate that stress. Then in 1998 a yoga studio opened up in the downtown area of Royal Oak, Michigan where I live. I started out with Ashtanga as I was in pretty good shape as a runner. Later that year I tried the more traditional yoga classes. I began to see some incredible benefits, which were so strong that in September of 2000 I decided to study to be a yoga teacher. I studied at Namaste Yoga. under Veronica Zador; by August 2001 I had my RYT (Registered Yoga Teacher with Yoga Alliance) certificate. Veronica is an extremely gifted shala (classes addressed to the study of yoga) and yoga class teacher as well as an incredible human being.

From Veronica, I learned how to plan a class very well and execute it. After I completed my studies, I was blessed once more and had the privilege of learning class design and actual teaching under my mentor Dawn Priebe, Dawn has an incredible gift with these. My style was very rigid in the beginning, but with much work, Dawn helped me to actually free associate a whole class. I am very grateful to her for this. During this period I went through the basic methods of copying other people's styles and trying them out, cutting and pasting as I went along. This brought me a long way and I learned important tools; however, I became frustrated because I did not know how to better assemble the wealth of knowledge I had attained from my teacher training. I found myself using only a small fraction of that information. I wanted to be able to dredge this information, and crystallize it into a class. Therefore, the next question I posed to myself was: "How do I create a class that has a certain focus and intention, while leveraging as much information as I can from my shala studies?"

My solution to this was to create a yoga class design template (see Figure 0.1). It has an arrangement of empty boxes and three basic sections. The first is comprised of sections "a" through "f," which are general preparation guidelines. The second is the body of the document, comprised of sections "g" through "o" , which define the postures and the qualities that these must meet based on your requirements. The third, section "p," or the closing section, concerns itself with moving into shavasana, the awakening dialog, and the closing dialog. The method of filling in this template will be discussed in detail in chapters 7 and 8. It is practical to use the results from the template directly or you can use it as a skeletal outline, free-associating on those ideas to create the class. Either of these extremes or any degree in between are all valid.

I finally decided to put all of this information into book form, mostly due to the encouragement from Veronica Zador.

0.2 From a High Level How Does This Book Work

In general, this book does not describe or list actual poses one might assemble for class. You will need to use other sources to acquire that information. A wealth of sources are available on that topic; and having your favorite sources available while reading this text is recommended. You will find them particularly useful as you work through chapters 7 and 8, in which you create the actual design of your class.

a) The main point and focus of this book are growth and reinvention. It's a way to break out and try something new and exciting
b) Stresses the use of fundamental, intermediate and advanced methods
c) Keeps all of the important information at your fingertips
d) Integrates a great deal of information
e) The tools presented are independent of class subject type (back class, abdominal strength etc)
f) The tools presented apply to all teaching styles ranging from free associated to analytically planned

g) It offers many ways of modifying your current teaching style

h) Helps you design a class from scratch with a specific purpose

i) Invent a different teaching style for yourself

j) Invent totally new types of classes

k) Create smaller flows to mix and match to create your class

l) Use any one concept in the book as an individual entity

m) Use combinations of concepts

n) Use the book as a handy reference for yoga class design

o) Chapters 1 through 6 provide a lot of individual concepts

p) Chapter 7 defines "The Class Design Template," that can be used to organize and integrate the data in chapters 1 through 6 into a class

q) Chapter 8 will give you 23 different graduated methods on how to use the text and template. These methods range from very easy to very difficult

r) When you become proficient you should be able to sketch up a new class in 10 to 15 minutes

s) You can also spend allot of time and go into great detail designing classes with this method

t) This text provides a foundation for and methods of growth throughout your teaching career

0.3 Introduction to Chapter 7 Basic Template Functionality

Don't get bogged down in this section. If it is not making sense you can always come back to it later.

The class design template shown in Figure 0.1 below is a structure designed by the author to help integrate the components presented in chapters 1 through 6. An introduction to the template and general usage is described in Fig 0.1 below. Boxes "a" through "f" and column "n" define information that gives general comments on how the class will be conducted. Column "g" defines the pose categories like, standing, sitting, inversions and so on. Letters "h," "i" and "j" refer to three separate curves that will be sketched in the tall column box below them. Letter "h" defines the effort level and will be represented by a solid line curve. Letter "i" refers to the stretch level curve and will be represented by dashed line curve. Lastly, letter "j" defines the speed level of the postures in your class and is represented by a dotted line curve. See figures 7.1.3 and 8.1.1 for examples of these. The boxes 1 through 48 in section "o" are for sketching actual postures or writing in the posture names for your class. Letters "k," "l" and "m" refer to sections of the text that are used to help organize your postures in section "o". Box "p" is for closing poses and comments.

The steps 7, 8 and 10 (from Figure 1) below define some specific functionality of the template. This functionality is described in detail in Figure 0.2.

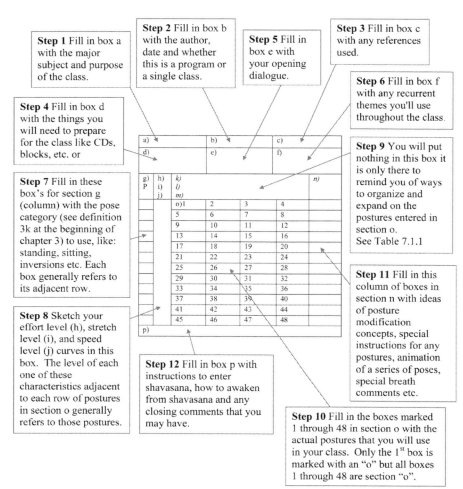

Step 1 Fill in box a with the major subject and purpose of the class.

Step 2 Fill in box b with the author, date and whether this is a program or a single class.

Step 5 Fill in box e with your opening dialogue.

Step 3 Fill in box c with any references used.

Step 4 Fill in box d with the things you will need to prepare for the class like CDs, blocks, etc. or

Step 6 Fill in box f with any recurrent themes you'll use throughout the class.

Step 7 Fill in these box's for section g (column) with the pose category (see definition 3k at the beginning of chapter 3) to use, like: standing, sitting, inversions etc. Each box generally refers to its adjacent row.

Step 9 You will put nothing in this box it is only there to remind you of ways to organize and expand on the postures entered in section o. See Table 7.1.1

Step 8 Sketch your effort level (h), stretch level (i), and speed level (j) curves in this box. The level of each one of these characteristics adjacent to each row of postures in section o generally refers to those postures.

Step 11 Fill in this column of boxes in section n with ideas of posture modification concepts, special instructions for any postures, animation of a series of poses, special breath comments etc.

Step 12 Fill in box p with instructions to enter shavasana, how to awaken from shavasana and any closing comments that you may have.

Step 10 Fill in the boxes marked 1 through 48 in section o with the actual postures that you will use in your class. Only the 1st box is marked with an "o" but all boxes 1 through 48 are section "o".

Figure 0.1 The Class Design Template Including General Definitions (see Figure 8.1.1 for a complete example)

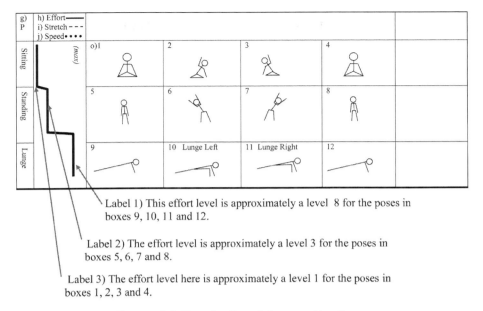

Label 1) This effort level is approximately a level 8 for the poses in boxes 9, 10, 11 and 12.

Label 2) The effort level is approximately a level 3 for the poses in boxes 5, 6, 7 and 8.

Label 3) The effort level here is approximately a level 1 for the poses in boxes 1, 2, 3 and 4.

**Figure 0.2 How to Read Across the Rows
of the Class Design Template**

Figure 0.2 is a general example of how the information described in steps 7, 8, and 10 (in figure 0.1) relate to one another. I am presenting these concepts here because they are probably the most complex within the book. If you understand these concepts up front, the rest of the book should be easy. If they are not clear after reading this section do not worry; we will cover this material in detail in several other areas of the book.

Definitions of nomenclature in Figure 0.2

Note the words "*min*" and "*max*": these describe levels for effort, stretch and speed. This span is broken down into ten levels where *min* = level 0 and *max* = level 10. In this case, I am restricting this explanation to the concept of effort. A max level of 10 would be the the maximum effort to you would ever expose a student to in the type of class you are designing. Note that Effort curves are represented by a solid line as shown in the legend. And, effort curves are definition "h" in the template. The thick solid stepped line sketched above refers to the effort level that we wish to use. Label 1 refers to a section of the effort curve that is about a level 8 out of 10. Label 2 points to a section of the curve that is about a level 3 and label 3 points to a section that is about a level 1. You can make your curves smooth or stepped as shown above.

Now we have enough definition to show how this process works. The first thing to do is to sketch in the effort level that you desire for the type of class you will be designing. Next, decide on the general pose progression you'll use throughout your class. Write the names of those general types in column "g". In the example above we have decided on sitting, standing, and lunge poses. The next step is to fill in the actual poses. You can either put a sketch of the pose or the actual pose name in each box. So in the boxes in section "o" marked 1 through 4, we want some seated poses that require only about a level 1 (or 10 percent of the maximum effort). In the second row, we want a series of standing postures that require about a level 3 (or 30 percent of the maximum effort). And in the next row, we want a series of lunges that require approximately a level 8 (or 80 percent of the maximum effort level). Labels 1, 2, and 3 also help illustrate this concept. If we were designing a class we would continue to form these relationships for the remaining rows of the template. Or, you may just use as many rows as appropriate for your class.

The relationships between the pose progressions described in column "g," the curves "h," "i" and "j," and the actual

poses are not intended in any way to be discreet or exact. These relationships are put there strictly as a mechanism to gain more control over your class design. The relationships are loosely associated and approximate. Therefore, major deviations are acceptable.

For example, a standing pose is acceptable in boxes 1 through 4. If somewhere in boxes 9 through 12 there happened to be an inversion that had an effort level of about 1 that's acceptable also. You could also sketch in several poses in each box if you needed to. Insert your information as desired to get your ideas into the template. I think you get the idea.

The same concepts described above also apply to the level of stretch and level of speed analogously. Note that when sketching in the level of stretch or speed, the lines are dashed and dotted respectively so you can distinguish them. The stretch level and speed levels are sketched in the same box that the effort level is shown in. If these concepts are not clear, don't worry; we will cover these concepts in detail in sections 4.10 and 4.11.

Now, what about when you actually use the ideas in the template to teach a class? Will you use them precisely as written? You can if you have sketched out a series of postures that define a reasonable flow. You could also just use the template as a skeletal outline. These concepts form two extremes. Any degree between these extremes is still a valid application.

On the lighter side of application maybe you only choose individual concepts within the text to apply occasionally and do not use the template at all. The degree to which you use these techniques is up to you.

0.4 Use and Benefits of the Class Design Template

a) Creates a standard format to document a yoga class
b) Keep a record of your classes for your own reference
(If you have each type of class that you teach documented, you can use those sheets to keep running records for improvements and modifications. This will help you grow as a teacher. There are many things that you may forget in the course of your career; if you keep your class design concepts documented you will be standing on a much larger knowledge base.)
c) **It will aid in your ability to integrate more techniques and information into one class**
(You will also find that both your class design skills and actual teaching techniques will improve. Since novel class designs are possible with these techniques you may find yourself developing new types of classes.)
d) Use it to share ideas with other teachers
e) Use it in formal training for other teachers
f) Use it to help teach students in special seminars
g) Use it to help document your personal research and development of your class style
h) Use it to document and conduct formal yoga research
i) Use it to take notes in shala. Note that if you do this, your notes will automatically be organized according to the sections of the template. This gives your notes a much greater value and makes them easier to read for future reference.
j) Use it to take notes in seminars

k) Use it to take notes while observing another teacher's class

l) Use it to collaborate with other teachers on yoga class design

m) Use it to develop and manage programs (a series of classes on the same subject matter)

n) Memorize the class you created in the template and teach it exactly as it is documented

o) Use the template just to get a rough idea on how the class should flow and teach from that reflection

p) Memorize only parts of the template and free-associate other parts

q) Use the template to document smaller flows that don't represent a whole class
    (Use these smaller flows to mix-and-match to create new classes.)

r) Use your template designs for job interviews

s) Design some core class types
    (You can then copy those sheets and modify them to create variations as desired.)

t) Two of the books cited in the endnotes "Anatomy of the Human Body" and "Anatomy and Human Movement" are two wonderful companion books for my book. Using the "Anatomy and Human Movement" text you can look up any joint in the body and determine its type and range of motion, muscles used etc. You can then look up the specific muscles and other core anatomy in "Anatomy of the Human Body".

0.5 My Writing Style

I will use the word "component(s)" to refer to the material presented in chapters 1 through 6. This could refer to the whole body of that information or any subset.

My general writing style will be to first describe a set of components for yoga class design and then propose ways of assembling the components. I cover this assembly process in chapter 7; it is a highly organized process. Some chapters include a set of definitions at the beginning of the chapter. These are included to help solidify the foundation of this text.

I intend to keep the idea development within this text as concise as possible. I want to be able to get the ideas across without embedding them in lengthy stories. This will serve to make the text easier to reference. The main component topics will be broken down into separate paragraphs which will be organized by: type, logical sequences, mode of application, degree, or function. Also, notice that each paragraph is numbered to aid in separation and referencing the concepts.

The chapter paragraph numbering uses a three number system like "3.1.2" The first number "3" refers to chapter 3. The "1" refers to the first subheading in chapter 3. The third digit "2" refers to sub-paragraphs under subheading "1."

Note that at the beginning of some of the chapters you will find a series of definitions. All definitions are listed in italic text. Definitions are numbered as follows, "*3a Program.*" The "3" refers to the chapter number and the letter "a" refers to the order in which the definition falls within that chapter. If there are subclassifications to definition 3a they will be followed with a number like "*3a1 Program Series.*" The numeral "1" in this case defines the first subclassification to definition 3a.

Also note that while taking notes and referring to this text you can easily refer to a definition by its label like "*3a1.*" You can also use the paragraph numbers like "3.1.3" to easily refer to sections in the book.

The basic focus of this book is for Hatha yoga teachers. Chapter 8 describes a series of graduated application methods of the template. This was included to make the text practical for as many different teaching styles and discipline levels as possible. There are six major levels ranging from beginner, intermediate, advanced intermediate, advanced, expert and advanced expert. These major levels have several sub levels. Each sub level is broken down into a series of steps that the teacher can follow. Each sub level addresses the concept of yoga class design from a different perspective.

<u>From an educational perspective the more different ways you learn to do a task the more advanced you will become at it and the deeper you will understand it.</u>

I created the methods and processes described in this book partly by using heuristic tools. The study of heuristics is one of my hobbies. Heuristics can mean many things; in general it seeks to define methods of discovery. Heuristic tools are also concerned with the way information is organized.

Information can take on a whole other character and meaning simply by the way it is arranged and organized. You may see more connections; you may understand the concepts more thoroughly. This gives you a significant advantage in making connections between ideas and seeing applications that may have been overlooked before. The study and practice of yoga has many esoteric components that are easily misplaced and or forgotten / left out once you form your initial style. The wealth and breadth of a yoga class is often dependent on being aware of and using these components where appropriate. This also gives you more control over how the class is designed. I am hoping that the teachers will find new and exciting class designs.

Here are four ways to apply this text:

1) Any single component presented in the book can be individually selected out for application into your class. Or you can pick out groups of components (remember components refers to the information presented in chapters 1 through 6). When considering the possible combinations of components presented, there are many possibilities. It is up to you to pick and choose and apply.

2) Learn how to insert the components into the template. This gives you a structured approach of applying the components to your class design. You can follow the general guidelines in chapter 7 and create your own process of using the template.

3) Pick out a few methods in chapter 8 to master.

4) Apply the graduated methods in chapter 8 from the beginning and do as many as you can. These methods hit the application of the template from many different angles. Your ability to create classes will then reach new levels. Your classes will also become much richer and dimensional because you will have packed them with much more information.

I present the more important ideas in three or four very different ways in an attempt to adequately define these concepts.

Within this text I am calling to your inner genius. You may not believe that the greatest of human potential takes residence within your soul, but everybody has the divine spark. I believe this and wish to inspire you to levels that you may have never imagined. Therefore, you will find no portion of this text that is "dumbed down"; I would never insult you. The intention here is to encourage you to grow in ways you may not think possible. This is the primary voice throughout this whole text. I hope the whole of this work resonates with each reader in that capacity and charges you with your own divinity.

Realize that the degree to which you change, reinvent, and grow has an edge in the same way that stretching a muscle does. So please consider the strength of your current foundation, your tolerance level for change, and the rate of change to which you subject yourself. Attempting to usher in too much change too quickly can be destructive. If you learn to manage these aspects and establish healthy limits you will keep yourself protected as you grow and shine.

0.6 How to Read This Book

One should approach chapters 1 through 6 with an attitude to gain a fair familiarization of the components. You may wish to take notes so you can remember the areas that are important to you.

Chapter 7 introduces the Class Design template. Read this chapter thoroughly and refer back to previous chapters were necessary.

Chapter 8 gives twenty-three graduated methods on how to use the template. Skim this chapter and find some techniques that you would like to try and then go back and follow the instructions for those specific application techniques.

I hope you find as much discovery, insight, and inspiration as I enjoyed while creating this work. Enjoy!

0.7 Contributors

The major contributors to my practice and this book are:

Veronica Zador, my shala teacher, made the process of studying nothing short of sheer joy. Not only did I learn the art and practice of yoga from her, but as an added benefit I found that my personal growth improved significantly during this period. After I showed Veronica some ideas I had been working on for yoga class design she inspired me to write this text. Veronica was also invaluable in helping to create the first rough outline of what the text would look like. After seven or eight drafts we finally came up with an image that seemed to work. Veronica also helped to edit the intermediate stages of the book. I am blessed to have crossed paths with Veronica and my life is permanently enriched for the honor of knowing her.

Dawn Priebe agreed to be my advisor and mentor in the application of teaching yoga. How lucky I am to have found another gifted person who was so supportive and giving during this process. Dawn somehow got me to move from a very inhibited approach of teaching to being able to free associate a whole class. There is really no way to repay such a valuable gift; I can only pay it forward. I will also forever cherish the discussions that we had after class about the practice and benefits of yoga. Dawn also helped in editing the text and had several significant insights that were included in reference to the edge. If I can quote her in reference to the long term practice of yoga: "It just keeps getting better!"

June and Lindsay, Proofreaders:

June Hayes was invaluable in the detailed editing of this text. I have known June for several years and have a deep respect and admiration for her teaching style. Therefore, I asked her if she would be so kind as to help me edit this work. She graciously agreed. Somehow, I managed to stumble upon a professional proofreader. If that is not karmic I don't know what is. June combed over and corrected what needed attention. June's attention to detail for syntax, grammar, and clarity are highly valued and much appreciated.

Lindsay Cole was extremely helpful in lending comments about application as she was the first one to pilot some of these ideas in her yoga class. Because I attend her class regularly, I was able to get feedback from her on some of the points of application. She also had several suggestions on how to make the template better, for which I am grateful and have included in its design. Lindsay further contributed by helping to proofread the whole text, from which many comments were included.

It has been an honor to work with these beautiful, intelligent individuals. Thank you!

0.8 Yoga Teacher Legacy

I want to extend a very special thank you to those inspired luminaries who invented, developed and carried on this tradition for thousands of years so that we may benefit.

1.0 Class Preparation and Opening Dialog

1.1 Self Preparation

1.1.1 Your grooming and clothing should be neat, clean, and not distracting. Consider how you are feeling that day: Is your mood up or down? This will have an effect on the class. The tone of your voice is also important; speaking from your heart will insure that you reach theirs. Lastly, your intention and why you're teaching will color everything. If you can bring your inspiration and share it, each word you utter will charge the air.

1.2 Room Issues

1.2.1 The students will notice as you are scurrying about, setting up things for their benefit. This helps to create a sacred space. In general the concept of room preparation should be to minimize distraction and create a soothing environment. Use incense or oils very lightly or not at all (ask the students first).

1.2.2 Adjust the heat and or air-conditioning if need be. In general keep the room warmer rather than cooler, as heat tends to open the body. If there are windows you might consider opening them to let in a cool breeze. Humidity is very important, because when people are taking deep breaths, dry air can be irritating to the throat. Good humidity levels are between 40 and 60 percent.

1.2.3 Adjust the lighting in the room so it is comfortable for the students. If there is direct sunlight coming in you might want to consider drawing the drapes to decrease the intensity. Use the actual lighting in the room to your advantage. A dimmer switch is great to custom-tailor the lighting to your class. Depending on what type of class you are conducting, consider that brighter rooms are more stimulating and darker ones are more relaxing. To create an even more spiritual experience, use candles in a dark or dimly lit room.

1.2.4 Clean floors and clean mats are essential.

1.2.5 I have always been a little up in the air about the use of music in yoga classes. One of the main purposes of yoga is to focus in on your internal palette. Any type of outside stimulation will tend to draw you away from that. But on the other hand, let's admit it, music can be lighthearted and fun.

1.2.6 If you have mirrors in the class against one wall arrange the students so their backs are towards the mirrors. This will keep the students from looking around too much. Yoga is a very internal practice so minimizing distractions is beneficial.

This also holds true for windows where distractions are present. However, if the windows are letting in something beautiful you may choose to focus the students towards that.

1.3 Student Issues

1.3.1 If you have several new students in a class you may wish to group them together so that when you provide special instruction all can benefit at the same time. You also might encourage them to sit in the front of the class so they can see better. This can be difficult because new students tend to be shyer and may want to sit in the back.

1.3.2 If you find yourself teaching a class with only a few students, consider arranging them in a circle or other unique arrangement. Fewer students in the class also lends itself to doing classes against the wall.

1.3.3 If you tend to have a class that is crowded you may want to consider staggering the mats. This way if you are doing sun salutations or other similar postures the students will not bump into one another.

1.3.4 If you will be using props, such as blocks, straps, blankets, or bolsters, ask the students to get those at the beginning of the class so that the class is not interrupted.

1.4 Actual Dialogue

1.4.1 One of the first things in establishing the opening dialog is to ask if anybody has anything actively healing in their body (or you can ask each student privately before the class starts). If they do have an injury but are unwilling to talk about it, let them know they should take care to protect that part of their body. In short, nothing should hurt. This naturally leads into the idea of the edge. Most of the time and for most classes its meaning is based on muscle stretching. The limit is described as the threshold of pain; you should be generally operating just below that. We will discuss this in depth in chapter 5.[1]

1.4.2 Creating a sacred space for your class is a challenge. This may involve revealing your own inspiration for teaching, what it means to you, and how you use that in the class. You might also like to share your stories of the benefits that you have realized through practicing yoga.[1]

1.4.3 The opening dialog should also center the students by helping them let go of their outside commitments and thoughts. Then, lead them to their internal space of body sensations and emotions. In essence, shift them from an external focus to an internal one. As this internal focus is established, give the students some tools to deal with this palette. One of the classic treatments is to encourage the students to allow whatever comes up to simply arise and pass. Another way I have heard this described is to act as an objective observer to one's own emotions. I also like to suggest that they can stop doing the directed poses and sit quietly or in child's pose. You may also consider giving them permission to leave the room and walk around a little outside of the class if things get too intense.[1]

1.4.4 Bring in your special perspective on the physiology of the body and how you perceive it to work. Many yoga instructors will find themselves with unique insights after long-term practice. Share this knowledge with your students.

1.4.5 There are many everyday applications of yoga. One of the most important revolves around the breath. In yoga you are encouraged to back off of the intensity of the pose whenever your breath becomes compromised. This will allow your breath to come back to its full and natural state. If this mechanism becomes second nature you may find yourself applying it in everyday life. In other words whenever anything you are doing, physically or mentally, causes your breath to become shallow or held, back off of that activity until your breath returns to a full deep state. I believe this to be one of the purposes of this mechanism.

1.4.6 If you have a tendency to be poetic or spiritual, go there with your voice. If it inspires you it will inspire your students.

1.4.7 Bring any other facet you can think of, be creative, reinvent yourself, apply those things that you always wanted to but were to shy about.

1.5 Recurrent Themes

1.5.1 Recurrent Themes for the Students
There are facets of a yoga practice that you may consider bringing up recursively. For example:
- reminding the students of how to breathe
- encouraging them to let go of their ego
- reflecting on the echo of a posture
- letting outside thoughts arise and pass

- concentrate on the posture sensations
- reminding them about their edge
Etc.

1.5.2 Recurrent Themes for the Teacher

The yoga instructor may also want to remind him or herself to:

- keep descriptions accurate
- make sure that students have a moment of silence every now and then
- make sure that an injured or compromised student is being adequately cared for
- don't give too much information
Etc.

The most important thing is the topic of the next chapter: the breath.

2.0 The Breath

"generally, The air received into
and expelled from the lungs
in the act of respiration.
to draw breath:
to inhale air,
breathe;
hence,
to live:
..." [2]

The purpose of this chapter is to describe the basics of the breathing mechanism and some of the metrics that affect its efficiency. I will also discuss the qualities of air that affect its oxygen content thus determining the oxygenation of the body. This section is included to build a foundation and strategy to manage breath issues. Therefore, if included in the template they will show up as reference notes.

2.0.1 Opening Dialogue

One of the purposes of the opening dialog should be to prepare the students to become aware of and work with their breath . The breath is the foundation of Hatha yoga, and it should remain constant and full throughout the whole class. Below you will find a breakdown of some of the facets of the breath.[1]

2.0.2 Breath Introduction

The actual breath is the invisible mass or volume of air that is inhaled and exhaled. The actual air cannot be seen. We can only experience it by sensations and the physical act of breathing. It is quite amazing how this most ethereal and delicate creature is also the most powerful to a yoga practice.

2.1 The Respiratory Tract

2.1.1 The nasal passages and sinuses have a mucous membrane, which aids in filtering and humidifying the air.[3]

2.1.2 The end of the nasal cavity connects to the pharynx, which has dual passages: one to the trachea and the other to the esophagus.[4]

2.1.3 The passageway to the lungs starts at the larynx. The larynx has an epiglottis flap-like structure. This flap closes when we swallow to keep any food or liquids out of the lungs.[5]

2.1.4 The larynx leads to the trachea (or windpipe), which splits into two passages called bronchi tubes. Each bronchi tube feeds a single lobe of the lungs.[6]

2.1.5 The bronchi are subsequently subdivided into smaller and smaller bronchial trees within each lung.

At the end of the bronchial trees are tiny elastic air sacs called alveoli. This is where most of the carbon dioxide and oxygen is exchanged. These alveoli form the main body of the lungs. The upper respiratory and bronchial passages are quite rigid compared to the alveolar walls. <u>During inhalation and exhalation the primary component of the breathing mechanism that actually expands and contracts to receive and expel the air are the alveolar sacs.</u>[6,7,8]

This mechanism is analogous to filling a balloon with a straw. The straw defines the passageway from the nasal cavities to the end of the bronchial tubes and the balloon defines the alveolar sac. Only the balloon expands and contracts; the straw remains relatively rigid. Alveoli are arranged like tiny bunches of interconnected balloons. These small structures massed together form the lobes of the lungs.

The number of alveoli in both lungs combined ranges from 274 to 790 million for the general population including male and female subjects. The mean number of alveoli is therefore just over 500 million. However, for the remainder of this text I am going to use 600 million because it is a nice round number for calculation purposes.[7,9]

2.2 The Muscles of Respiration

2.2.1 The primary muscle for inhalation during normal breathing is the diaphragm. The diaphragm is a horizontal muscle extending across the bottom of the rib cage. It also separates the thoracic from the abdominal cavity. The exhalation in this state is primarily due to this muscle relaxing and coming back to a neutral state.[10,11,12]

2.2.2 When employing a full breath the inhalation also activates the external intercostal muscles, which raise the lower ribs. The external intercostal muscles are attached to adjacent ribs. Also, the scalene and Sternocleidomastoideus (Sternomastoid muscle) expand the upper ribs and sternum. The scalene muscles (there are three on either side of the neck) are attached between the cervical vertebrae and the upper ribs. The sternomastoid muscles are attached between the sternum and clavicle at the bottom and the mastoid process of the skull on the top.[10, 12, 13,14,15]

2.2.3 During exhalation for this full breath the rectus and transverse abdominus, external obliques and the internal intercostal muscles become active. The rectus abdominus are attached between the lower ribs and the pubic symphysis. The transverse abdominus muscle operates horizontally in the torso, it has many connection points (too complicated to describe for the level of this text). The external oblique muscles exist in the same space as the transverse abdominus muscles but operate at an angle between the vertical and horizontal. The internal intercostal muscles attach between adjacent ribs and when they contract they pull the ribs together and down. These muscles aid in expiration by compressing the lower part of the thorax.[10, 12, 13,16]

2.2.4 In order to open up the breath, one might start by developing stretches for the breathing muscles described above. There are other muscles involved in the respiration process these are some of the major contributors.

2.3 How the Expansive and Contractive Forces are Transmitted from the Breathing Muscles to the Alveolar Sacs

2.3.1 During inhalation the thoracic cavity expands via the breathing muscles. Physically attached to the inner wall of the thoracic cavity is a thin membrane called the parietal pleura. This membrane also expands with the thoracic cavity. The surface of the lung is surrounded by another thin membrane called the visceral or pulmonary pleura. These membranes are attached at their edges and form a space that can hold fluid. If a section is cut in the transverse plane through the center of the thoracic cavity one would see that these membranes wrap around the lung for about 310 degrees. The approximate 50 degree section is open to accommodate the mediastinum. This is in general the area between the lungs that houses the heart, trachea, esophagus, and a host of vascular entities.[17]

2.3.2 The space between these pleural membranes is called the pleural cavity. The pleural cavity is filled with a fluid. This fluid creates cohesive forces which hold the two membranes together. These forces are the same as when you have a thin film of water between two plates of glass. You can slide them parallel to one another with little resistance; however, if you try to pull them apart by applying a force perpendicular to their surfaces it is very difficult to separate them. The lungs make use of both the free sliding action and the normal force transmission of this mechanical mechanism.[18]

2.3.3 This essentially means that as the breathing muscles expand and contract the thoracic cavity, they can apply a normal force to the surface of the lungs to expand and contract them also. The sliding action allows the lungs to expand and contract freely and smoothly so that they are not stressed or damaged in the process. This free expansion also allows the alveolar sacs to expand in a uniform and symmetric manner. If the alveolar sacs were not allowed to expand uniformly, it would create additional stress in their delicate tissues.

To exemplify this picture a standard rubber balloon that has been inflated. If you want to damage the balloon all you have to do is grab one side of it and squeeze. By squeezing the balloon you are simulating a nonuniform expansion. This creates high stresses in the balloon wall and may cause it to pop. If you leave the balloon alone so its expansion is uniform the stresses in the walls will be much lower. This is the purpose of the fluid in the pleural cavity which allows for the uniform expansion of the lungs and minimizes the stresses in the alveolar sacs.

2.3.4 To summarize: the actual force mechanism begins with the breathing muscles expanding the thoracic cavity. The parietal pleura is connected to the thoracic cavity and expands with it. The fluid in the pleural cavity creates a cohesive force that holds the visceral pleura to the parietal pleura. This is why the visceral pleura expands with the parietal pleura. The visceral or pulmonary pleura is directly connected to the alveolar sacs which comprise the wall of the lung. Therefore, the lung (alveolar sacs) will expand as the visceral pleura expands. This action is allowed to happen in a relatively stress-free uniform manner because of the sliding action of the pleural cavity between the two membranes.

2.4 How the Expansion and Contraction of the Alveolar Sacs Moves the Air

2.4.1 The expansion of the lungs creates an increase in volume and relative drop in pressure which forces air through the breathing channel described above into the alveolar sacs. When the lungs contract, they create an increase in pressure which forces air out of the lungs.[19]

2.4.2 To continue with the example above we can now place the balloon inside of a bellows, then connect the straw to the mouth of the bellows. Here the bellows represent the thoracic cavity and the breathing muscles activate the bellows. During inhalation the breathing muscles expand the bellows and the balloon inside (alveolar sac) expands drawing in air.

2.4.3 As the diaphragm and intercostal muscles contract, the thoracic cavity--and thus the alveolar sacs—contract, causing a decrease in volume. This causes an increase in pressure inside the alveolar sacs which forces air out of the lungs. (This mechanism is directly analogous to squeezing a baloon to force air out of it. If there is a narrow opening you can feel the air rushing out.)[12]

2.4.4 Proceeding with the analogy, during exhalation the breathing muscles contract the bellows along with the balloon inside (alveolar sac) pushing the air out.

2.4.5 Now that we have developed the breathing mechanism this far, let's extend the argument. Instead of one balloon (alveolar sac) inside of the bellows let's visualize many very small ones. As the bellows is expanded and contracted each of the smaller sacs is expanded and contracted also, just like the single large balloon. The mechanism is similar.

2.5 Application of This Mechanism to Breathing Exercises

"…..Sealing in little thuribles dreams and wisdom,
Incense beyond all price, forever fragrant,
A breath whereof makes clear the eyes of the soul!
How I inhaled its sweetness……" [20]

2.5.1 Now let's think about breathing by only expanding the lower part of the thoracic cavity. If this is done the small balloons (alveolar sacs) in that region will expand and contract. By expanding different parts of the thoracic cavity we can see that this will primarily cause the relative alveolar sacs in the expanded region to draw in air.

2.5.2 This might start to sound familiar to anyone who has done the three-part yoga breathing exercise. This exercise starts by expanding the lower thoracic cavity then proceeds to expand the middle and then the upper thoracic cavity. So what this exercise strives to achieve is to expand and contract all of the alveolar sacs in the lungs. This results in a very full breath. The health benefits of this are that we regularly exercise all (or a majority) of the alveolar sacs.[1]

2.5.3 The exhalation is done in the reverse order by collapsing the upper thoracic cavity then the middle and then the lower.

2.6 The Volume of the Alveolar Sacs

The values in the arguments presented below are reasonably close for an adult male. Some values were rounded off for ease of calculation.

2.6.1 After a maximum inhalation to the total lung capacity each alveoli is about 0.267 mm in diameter. In this state the volume of each alveolar sac is roughly 0.010 mm^3. Remember we decided to use the value of 600 million alveoli in both lungs combined. With these values the total volume of the alveolar sacs (or lungs) at full inhalation would be about 6.0 L.[9, 21]

2.6.2 At the time of maximum exhalation to the residual volume each alveoli is about 0.147 mm in diameter. The volume of each alveolar sac at this time is roughly 0.00167 mm^3. The residual volume is the minimum amount of air that your lungs can hold. The total volume of the alveolar sacs at this time is roughly 1 L of air.[21]

2.6.3 If your lungs were in a neutral state, as they would be in a cadaver, the diameter of each alveoli would be roughly 0.20 mm. The volume of each alveolar sac at this time is roughly 0.0042 mm^3. The total volume of the alveolar sacs at this time is roughly 2.50 L of air.[21]

2.6.4 The difference between the fully expanded volume of 6.0L and the residual volume of 1.0L is equal to 5.0L of air. This defines the vital capacity or the maximum volume of air that your respiratory tract can pass with each inhalation or exhalation. The general term for lower volumes of fresh air entering and leaving the lungs are "tidal volumes." The amount of air left in the lungs after a tidal volume exhalation is called the functional residual capacity.[21]

2.6.5 For comparison purposes, the tidal volume that we use during normal daily activity is about 0.5L. This is only about 10% of the vital capacity. Therefore, during normal activity we are using a very small amount of our lung capacity.[21]

2.6.6 The anatomical dead space within the respiratory system is defined as the volume of the air passages beginning at the inlet of the nose to the inlet of the alveolar sacs. From our previous example this would be the volume of the straw. For this example, let's begin with the exhalation. At the end of the exhalation we can clearly see that the dead space is still full of exhaled air. This means that the first part of the next inhalation will be the dead space volume of this exhaled air. This volume is approximately 0.15 L of air; but for calculation and example purposes I will round this off to 0.2L. Therefore, the actual volume of fresh air entering the lungs will be the tidal volume (or vital capacity) minus the dead space.[22, 21]

2.7 Breath Investigation

Since the mechanism of breathing has been basically laid out it will be interesting to study the effects of deeper inhalations and exhalations. I would like to demonstrate which is more efficient, a deeper inhalation or exhalation. With the knowledge presented in prior sections and the conditions given below this demonstration can be expressed as an engineering problem.

Assumptions / Conditions:

1) We will assume that the lungs are 100% efficient and all processes and mechanisms are uniform and homogeneous.
2) This investigation was conducted analytically; no subjects or measurement equipment was used.
3) All volumes presented below are reasonably within the size range of actual anatomical structures.
4) We will assume that the air representing the functional residual capacity and dead space air have negligible oxygen content.
5) The tidal volume is increased to the same value for the greater inhalation and exhalation.

There will be three cases presented: Case I which is the control case, Case II which represents the deeper inhalation and Case III that represents the deeper exhalation. In Case II and Case III the deeper inhalations and exhalations are equivalent so as to be comparable.

2.7.1 Case I - (see Table Below): This case starts with a functional residual capacity of 2.0L and our individual inhales a tidal volume of 0.5L. Of this 0.5L the first 0.2L is dead space air and the remaining 0.3L is fresh air. The total volume of the lungs in this case is the functional residual capacity of 2.0L + the tidal volume of 0.5L = 2.5L of air. The percent of fresh air in the lungs in this case is 12 % (or 0.3 / 2.5 * 100).

2.7.2 Case II: Case II starts with the same functional residual capacity of 2.0L, but here our individual inhales more deeply to a tidal volume of 1.0L. Of this 1.0L the first 0.2L is dead space air, and the remaining 0.8L is fresh air. The total volume of the lungs in this case is the functional residual capacity of 2.0L + the tidal volume of 1.0L = 3.0L of air. The percent of fresh air in the lungs is now 26.67 % (or 0.8 / 3.0 * 100).

2.7.3 Case III: In the last case our individual begins by exhaling more deeply to a functional residual capacity of 1.5L. Then our individual inhales to the same tidal volume of 1.0L. Of this 1.0L the first 0.2L is dead space air and the remaining 0.8L is fresh air. The total volume of the lungs in this case is the functional residual capacity of 1.5L + the tidal volume of 1.0L = 2.5L of air. The percent of fresh air in the lungs in this case is 32.0 % (or 0.8 / 2.5 * 100).

2.7.4 In conclusion, under the conditions given above the deeper exhalation is more efficient in oxygenating the lungs. Case III is 5.33% more efficient than case II. Note that this is true even though the amount of fresh air in the lungs is the same for both the greater inhalation of case II and the greater exhalation of case III. The reason this efficiency difference occurs is because the functional residual capacity is reduced in case III by taking a greater exhalation. This in effect reduces the starting volume of the lungs, then, by taking in the same volume of fresh air the concentration of oxygen is increased. This may be one of the reasons that a prolonged exhalation is encouraged in some yoga practices.

All values in the table below are in liters.

	Functional Residual Capacity	Tidal Volume	Dead Space	Fresh Air Volume	Total Lung Volume	% Of Fresh Air In Lungs
I) Normative Case	2.0	0.5	0.2	0.3	2.5	12.00
II) Fuller Inhale	2.0	1.0	0.2	0.8	3.0	26.67
III) Fuller Exhale	1.5	1.0	0.2	0.8	2.5	32.00

Table 2.7.1 Breath Investigation

2.8 Qualities of Air

2.8.1 Relative humidity is the relative amount of water vapor in the air. Water vapor displaces air molecules, therefore the more humid the air is the less oxygen content it will have.[23]

2.8.2 Air density refers to how tightly packed the air molecules are. An increase in pressure will cause the air molecules to become more tightly packed thus increasing the air and oxygen density. For example, the top of Mount Everest is roughly 9,145 m (30,000 feet) above sea level. The air pressure at this altitude is roughly 30,340 Pa (4.4 psi). Since this is a relatively low-pressure (compared to where most people live) the air density and oxygen content will also be low and it will be harder to breathe. The Dead Sea is roughly 455 m (1,500 feet) below sea level. The air pressure at this altitude is roughly 106,870 Pa (15.5 psi). Since this is a relatively high-pressure the air density will also be higher.[23]

2.8.3 Increasing the temperature of air will also decrease its density; therefore it will have a lower oxygen content.[23]

2.8.4 Air quality is an issue since particulate matter and the presence of polluting gasses will also displace oxygen molecules making it harder to breathe.

2.8.5 Normal air composition is roughly 21% oxygen and 78% nitrogen. The remaining 1% other naturally occurring gasses. [24] In general the denser the air is the easier it will be to breathe. This is true because as the air becomes denser the density of oxygen will increase also (the opposite is true also). Reference 23 cited in this section gives an equation of air density as a function of temperature pressure and the amount of water vapor or humidity (and other values). It is found that pressure is directly proportional so that as the pressure increases so will the density. Temperature is found to be inversely proportional so as the temperature increases the density will decrease. The term for the amount of water vapor in the equation is found to be a negative; therefore as the humidity increases its term will become more negative and it will decrease the density of the air. This is the basis upon which the arguments in sections 2.8.1 through 2.8.3 were arrived.

2.9 Breath Awareness

2.9.1 Awareness of the breath by simply observing it is one of the most basic breath exercises. This is a fundamental step in the journey to create a relationship with your breath. As it is written or spoken it sounds simple or trivial, but make no mistake: it can be extremely difficult. It is important not to push ourselves too quickly into this. The inward journey should be accompanied by a sense of honor and patience. [1]

2.10 The Sensations Caused by Breathing.

"A SIMPLE Child,
That lightly draws its breath,
And feels its life in every limb," [25]

The sensations caused by breathing have an interesting purpose in the scope of a yoga class. They aid in the student's potential to develop a relationship with their breathing. Listed below are ways to investigate these sensations.

2.10.1 Can you feel the sensation of your breath on your upper lip as you breathe through your nose? [1]

2.10.2 Can you feel the passage of air inside your nose and throat?

2.10.3 Can you hear the sound of your normal breath?

2.10.4 What is the temperature of the breath?

2.10.5 Is the breath dry or is it humid?

2.10.6 Can you visualize your breath?

2.10.7 Focusing on the physical movement is probably the easiest to perceive. This is because you can actually see and feel the breathing muscles and ribs expanding and contracting.

2.11 Relative Breath Expansion

What part of the body expands when breathing? Also investigate the order in which these areas expand.

2.11.1 Lower abdomen

2.11.2 Solar plexus

2.11.3 Chest

2.11.4 Upper back

2.11.5 Mid back

2.11.6 Lower back

2.12 Breath Channel

What is the channel by which your breath moves into and out of your body?

2.12.1 Inhaling and exhaling through your nose (it appears to be generally accepted that nose breathing has many benefits over mouth breathing). It cleans and humidifies the air and promotes slower breathing.

2.12.2 Inhaling and exhaling through your mouth.

2.12.3 Inhaling through your nose and exhaling through your mouth.

2.12.4 Inhaling through your mouth and exhaling through your nose.

2.12.5 Inhaling and exhaling through both your nose and mouth.

2.13 Lung Capacity[21] (some values rounded)

12.13.1 The vital capacity is the maximum volume of air that you are capable of breathing in (after your deepest exhalation to the residual volume) during one inhalation. This is about 5.0L of air for the average male.

12.13.2 Most exercise will have tidal volumes somewhere between 5.0L and 0.5L of oxygen.

12.13.3 The tidal volume used during normal daily activities is about 0.5L of air for the average male.

2.14 Breath Duration and Transitions

What is the duration of the inhale and exhale? You can measure this by counting the number of seconds it takes to inhale, then measure the number of seconds it takes to exhale.

2.14.1 Is the inhalation the same length as the exhalation?

2.14.2 Is the inhalation longer than the exhalation?

2.14.3 Is the exhalation longer than the inhalation?

2.14.4 What is the length of the transitional pause at the end of the inhalation?

2.14.5 What is the length of the transitional pause at the end of the exhalation?

2.15 Breath Rate (volume of air / second) of the Inhalation or Exhalation

"Smile, breathe and go slowly" [26]

2.15.1 Same rate from start to finish

2.15.2 Starts slow then gradually speeds up

2.15.3 Starts fast then gradually slows down

2.15.4 Starts slow increases rate then slows again

2.15.5 Starts fast then slows then increases again

2.16 What is the Breath Quality

2.16.1 Jerky and jagged

2.16.2 Smooth and easy

2.16.3 Much effort

2.16.4 Little effort

2.17 The Basic Relationship Between the Postures and the Breath

"All things bear the shade on their backs
And the sun in their arms;
By the blending of breath
From the sun and the shade,
Equilibrium comes to the world." [27]

2.17.1 One relationship between the postures and breath is that the breath should always remain constant, even though the postures challenge the consistency of the breath. This is one of the fundamental concepts in a yoga practice. More accurately stated: the expression of the postures should always be modified in order to keep the breath constant, smooth, and full. The breath comes first. The breath and heart rate will tend to increase with the level of difficulty of the pose. When you become taxed, the reaction may be to hold your breath. If either of these happens it is a signal for the student to decrease the intensity of the pose.[1]

3.0 Class Design Methods

3.0.1 Now that the breath and the relationship between the breath and postures has been established, the next challenge is to develop a series of postures that achieve your class subject. I will present some definitions followed by strategies for deriving the postures for your class.

Definitions:

Defining a Program

3a) Program
A program is a series of classes conducted in a certain order to create a desired effect on the students.

3a1) Program Series
The program series can be any length (three classes, ten classes, twenty classes etc).

3a2) Program Subject Matter
Program subject matter may include things like: strengthening, flexibility, emotional aspects, spiritual, back pain,

general relaxation, cardiovascular health, or some physical type of ailment. For example, your program subject could be to improve core strength. Here you could address the abdominal muscles, chest and shoulders and the back.

3a3) Program Subject Division

Subject division in general means to divide the scope of your subject matter into the number of classes that you have chosen. This is a process for defining the subject for each class within your program. For example, let's say you are designing a program with three classes and the subject of your program is to improve core strength. The next step would be to divide the subject matter into three classes. The first class might be designed to strengthen the abdominal muscles; the second class might work the chest and shoulders; the last class might be designed to strengthen the back.

Defining a Class

3b) Class Subject Matter

Class subject matter may include things like: strengthening, flexibility, emotional aspects, spiritual, back pain, general relaxation, cardiovascular health, or some physical type of ailment. If you are just designing a single class you will not use the program ideas above.

3c) Major Pose

Major poses are the core poses that are chosen to support the class subject. For example, if you are going to design a class for one of the specific subjects described above, you would select a series of major poses that create the desired effect on the body. A series of major poses can be used to design the whole class; however, while it will serve the purpose of supporting your subject it will probably not flow very well because there will be no introductory, counter, or transitional poses. Refer to the major pose expansion concepts (described below).

Major Pose Expansion Concepts:

3d) Test Poses and Other Testing Tools
A test pose(s) will help to determine where the student's edge is. Refer to chapter 5 for an explanation of the edge. This allows the teacher to adjust the level of difficulty (or some other facet) of the pose. You could evaluate the students flexibility edge by applying test poses that address the aspect of flexibility with which you are working. For example, if you plan to use many deep forward folds in your class, use a forward fold as a test pose. While the class is executing this pose, observe each student closely. If the students have no difficulty with the depth of the test pose then you can probably proceed as planned. If however, you perceive a few students who have great difficulty, you may wish to consider modifying the depth of the fold. You could also only adjust those few individuals who are having trouble.

If you are planning to do a long meditation later in the class, first test to see if they can at least sit with their eyes closed. If these students can't even sit with their eyes closed, then certainly you would not sit them for a long meditation. If they can, then maybe try a one-minute meditation to see if anybody gets uncomfortable. If they succeed you can probably proceed to the longer meditation. In this example, I am suggesting that you can apply more and more difficult tests to see where your audience is.

Prior to working with a series of difficult strengthening poses you may wish to introduce some strength-based test poses. This means to test the strength of the class in the muscle groups that you are going to be working. As the class executes these test poses, watch them very carefully for signs of fatigue. Adjust the difficulty of these poses to suit the class.

Chanting "om" is a way to evaluate the energy level of the class, albeit a rough one. The only way to really understand this is to ask the students how they are feeling. You could begin the class with an om and listen to the intensity. Test again in the middle of the class to see the effect that your poses are having. Are they getting stronger or are they running out of energy? Use this reaction to determine how to proceed. Also, listen for the duration or how long they are capable of holding the om. This may be an indication of how deep the breath of the class is likely to be. It is not the opinion of the author that this method is highly accurate. This is just an approximate technique.

Test poses are particularly useful to help evaluate new students and to help learn how hard to push your current students. Test poses can also be applied periodically throughout the class to evaluate where the students are at any one particular time.

Test poses are extremely useful and <u>very important to apply</u> when dealing with groups of people with special needs (see Chapter 6).

3e) Introductory Poses
Introductory poses are typically poses that are similar to the major pose but easier. They may even be the same pose

but a less deep expression of it. Introductory poses are used to warm up the major pose.[1]

3f) Counter Poses
Counter poses are poses that balance out the major pose. For example, a counter pose to a forward fold would be a backbend. A counter pose for headstand would be child's pose. Poses that are expressed left to right generally do not require a counter pose; this is because they inherently counter themselves.[1]

3g) Transitional Poses
Transitional poses are poses that create a smooth flow by connecting two dissimilar poses. For example if you wanted to move from plank pose to a standing forward fold you could use downward dog as a transitional pose. Downward dog in this case gets you half way there and makes the transition to the standing forward fold smoother.[1]

3h) Stretching Strengthening Sequences
In this case the major pose(s) simply needs to be found someplace within the sequence. Begin with a pose that stretches a certain muscle group. Follow immediately with a pose that strengthens that same muscle group. There are some poses that will both stretch and strengthen a muscle group at the same time. You can apply this recursively to create the whole class. Another strategy would be to apply these selectively in specific places within the class.[1]

These sequences might look something like:
- stretching pose 1, strengthening pose 1, stretching pose 2, strengthening pose 2 etc.

- strengthening pose 1, stretching pose 1, strengthening pose 2, stretching pose 2 etc.

3i) Multiple Pose Stretching Strengthening Sequences
Another strategy is to do a series of stretching exercises and then follow that with a series of strengthening exercises for those same muscle groups. For example, you might do five poses that stretch a certain muscle group followed by five poses that strengthen that group. Also in this case, the major pose(s) only needs to be found somewhere within the sequence.

These sequences might look something like:
- stretching pose 1, stretching pose 2, strengthening pose 1, strengthening pose 2, etc.
- strengthening pose 1, strengthening pose 2, stretching pose 1, stretching pose 2, etc.

3j) Closing Poses
Closing poses are a series of poses that are designed to transition the student into shavasana. These are typically poses on the back, such as knees into the chest with rocking or some spinal twists.[1]

Pose Grouping Concepts

3k) Pose Category
The pose category describes the general type of poses you are using. Some examples of pose categories are standing, sitting, inverted, on back etc. Within each pose category is a group of poses of that type.[28]

3l) Pose Progression

The pose progression is the order in which the categories are arranged from start to finish. For example, you may begin with seated, then move to standing, then inversions, etc. There are examples of pose progressions in classic yoga textbooks.

Pose Series Concepts

Note that any pose series can be used to organize the postures within a pose category. Also, any pose series described below can be used to define the whole class.

3m) Intentional Series of Poses

An intentional series of poses is primarily concerned with the relationship between the major poses that support your class subject. The major poses are ordered such that each successive pose has some beneficial and intentional relationship to the one preceding it. You can still use all of the other tools like introductory, counter, and transitional poses; they do not interfere with an intentional series.

For example if your class subject is to open up the spine, you could do this by using its six degrees of freedom. The poses could be something like: 1) forward fold, 2) backbend, 3) left side stretch, 4) right side stretch, 5) left side twist, 6) right side twist.

These would then represent your major poses because each one has a very specific and intentional relationship to the one preceding it. In the most general terms, this is because they all assist in opening up the spine. The front to back and lateral stretches help warm up the spine prior to doing the twists. You can embellish these major poses however you like with introductory, counter, and transitional poses, and so on.

3n) Contiguous Series of Poses
A contiguous series of poses are a group of poses that begin in one area of the body and gradually progress to another. For example, one contiguous series might begin at the feet and gradually progress to the head. In other words, this would mean to select a series of poses that begin by stretching the feet, then proceed to the calf muscles, the thighs, the hips, lower abdomen, middle abdomen, chest, neck, and, finally, the head.

Developing a contiguous series can be done in the following ways:
- Begin by opening up the breathing muscles and then move outward to other areas of the body.
- Begin at the head and move towards the feet.
- Begin at the feet and move towards the head.
- Begin at the core abdominal muscles and move outwards towards the limbs.
- Massage therapists, sometimes use the following sequence: begin with the upper back, then proceed down the torso to the feet, then proceed to the upper chest and move down the torso to the feet, then go to the shoulders and arms moving to the hands; lastly, provide stretches to the neck and head.

3o) Smooth Flow Series of Poses
A smooth flow series of poses are a group of poses that fit together very well. The transition between each one of these poses is very gradual. These transitions may also be

described as fluid and effortless. This type of series is not necessarily contiguous or intentional. The major pose expansion techniques can be used to help create a smooth flow series.

3p) General Series of Poses

A general series of poses is any preplanned group of postures; no other conditions apply. In other words, they are not necessarily intentional, contiguous, or smooth flow etc.

3q) Imitated Series of Poses

An imitated series of poses is a series of poses that is copied from a book or learned from another teacher. The whole class or any portion of it can be copied. Copying styles is probably one of the most effective ways of learning for the new teacher. You might try to analyze the series by breaking it down into major, counter, introductory, etc. You can also look for grouping and series concepts.

3r) Free Associated Series

A free associated series is a series of poses that is made up on the spot. No pre-planning at all is done. An interesting challenge is to free-associate an intentional series with a smooth flow.

3s) Combined Series of Poses

A combined series of poses employs any combination of these series techniques.

3t) Mix and Match Series

You can create standard sets of short series from any of the series definitions. Then mix and match the smaller series to create your class.

3u) Right and Left Hand Expression Series
As an added dimension you could also do a series of poses on the right side of the body then do the same series on the left. For example some poses have a natural right and left hand expression like triangle and warrior pose. To apply this technique you would first do both right hand expressions of these postures, followed by both left hand expressions.

3.1 General Considerations on the Class or Program Subject Matter

3.1.1 In general the subject should be selected to provide the maximum benefit to the students.

Every teacher has their strengths. The techniques provided in this text should allow the teacher to both build on their strengths and reinvent themselves in creative ways to improve in areas where they are not as experienced. You may want to design a certain type of class but are unsure as to how to go about it from scratch. This chapter provides many options for this process. First, refer to definitions 3a to 3c and decide how you will proceed. Will you be designing a program containing a series of classes, or will you just design one class? If you are designing a single class you can ignore all 3a definitions.

3.1.2 Set up a subject based on muscle groups. For example, if you're creating a program on strengthening, you might begin with strengthening the abdominal muscles, followed by the back for the next class, then maybe the chest muscles, then a class for the legs, and the last class might be to strengthen the arms. If you look at the sequence of classes you will see that there is a purpose behind the order. It began by strengthening the core of the body by first working the abdominal area then the back. Then move to the muscle groups that are more dependent on the core namely the legs and then lastly strengthening the arms. If you are designing a single class you can incorporate all or part of these ideas into one class. Use the same order but fewer postures to accommodate.

3.1.3 Set up a subject to address emotional states or physical conditions. Designing your class to affect the chakras or acupressure points is one way to do this.

3.1.4 Consider your audience. You may be dealing with a certain cross section of society that has specific issues. You could select a series of class subjects that address the general well-being of this group. Selecting some combination of subject matter that address the muscle groups, physical ailments, and emotional states of this group will serve your students well.

3.1.5 Social events may be very stressful at times, and at other times can be very calm and uneventful. Modify the subject of your yoga class accordingly. During very stressful times you may want to choose a class subject that is very gentle and nurturing. When things are more normal you may choose to push them more.

3.1.6 You should also consider the time of year. It is obvious to everyone that in the warmer months the body is more open and flexible; in the colder months, the opposite.

3.1.7 Provide a special treat for your students by designing special classes specifically for holidays and special events.

3.1.8 One of the most important subject considerations in your yoga class is in relation to your most challenged students. If you happen to find yourself teaching people with special needs the subject matter should be adjusted accordingly. Special consideration for the edge sensitivity within this group is important. See chapter 6 for more information on this topic.

3.2 Define Your Program

3.2.1 The first step in defining a program is to choose the subject matter (see section 3.1). Next, define the number of classes within it. Follow this by performing the program subject division (see definition 3a3). This is done by dividing the scope of your subject matter within the number of classes that you have chosen to conduct.

3.3 Define Your Class

3.3.1 The first step in defining a class is to choose the subject matter (see section 3.1).

3.3.2 Begin by selecting a series of major poses (definition 3c) that support the subject of your class. It creates the foundation to derive the other postures from. You could begin by selecting a series of postures that affect the muscle groups you wish to address. For example, if you were going to create a class to strengthen and stretch the lower back you would begin by selecting a series of major poses that affect the muscle groups in that area. You may wish to design a whole class that is focused around opening up the breathing muscles described in the previous chapter.

3.3.3 The major pose expansion definitions (3d through 3i) provide a systematic way of expanding your major poses into an actual class. Start with a major pose, put an introductory pose in front of it. After the major pose you can provide a counter pose. Follow the counter pose with a transitional pose to the next introductory pose. Continue this process through all of your major poses. The final sequence might look something like this:

introductory1, major1, counter1, transitional1, introductory2, major2, counter2, transitional2, …

These help to protect the class by warming up to each pose using introductory poses and moving smoothly to the next by using transitional poses. Apply counter poses where necessary. The strengthening and stretching sequences can also be used. Lastly, closing poses can be applied to transition to shavasana.

3.3.4 Major pose grouping concepts (*definitions 3k and 3l*) are useful and are also referenced in classical yoga textbooks. You essentially use these by organizing your postures into categories like: standing, sitting, inverted, etc. Then the categories are organized into a progression. Lastly, you can organize the poses within each category and develop them further using some of the major pose expansion concepts or pose series concepts.

3.3.5 Pose series concepts provide a wealth of approaches to class design. The pose series concepts can be used to define the whole class or any part of it. Refer to definitions 3m through 3u for pose series concepts.

3.4 Analyzing Other Teachers Series

3.4.1 The definitions provided in this chapter can be a useful tool to analyze groups of poses from other teachers. For example:

a) Can you find the class subject?
b) Based on the subject can you pick out the major poses of this group?
c) Can you identify the use of any of the major pose expansion techniques?
d) Can you find the presence of pose grouping concepts like categories and progressions?
e) Do any of the pose series concepts seem to be present?

This chapter presents the possibility for many different approaches to yoga class design and analysis. Enjoy!

4.0 Posture Modification Concepts

Posture modification concepts refer to things that you can do to a pose after you have established the breath and the basic shape of the core pose. This chapter describes some of the tools to modify a posture, but it does not address the boundaries and safety precautions required to keep the body properly aligned. It is up to the teacher to properly research and apply these concepts.

Definitions:

Major and Minor Modifications

4a) Major Modifications:
Major modifications to a pose are when you move a limb or the torso significantly out of the core pose. An example of a major modification would be raising one leg towards the ceiling while in downward dog.[1]

4b) Minor Modifications
Minor modifications deal more with subtle alignment and are measured in millimeters. A teacher can instruct on minor

modifications or the intuition of the student can bring them to light. The general concept is to make small modifications to the pose once you have entered it with the intention of making it feel better. An example of a minor modification would be to slightly vary the angle of a joint in order to make the posture feel better to you.[29]

Spatial Modifications:

4c) Abduction and Adduction
Abduction and adduction, respectively, mean to move any body part away from or towards (respectively) the center-line (imaginary line through the spine) of the body.[30,31,32]

4d) Pronation and Supination
Pronation refers to rotating the feet to the inside. Putting more weight onto the big toe side of the foot is a pronation. Supination is the opposite motion: rotating the feet to the outside, putting more pressure on the small toe side of the foot.[31, 33,34,35]

4d1) Forearm Pronation and Supination
Pronation and Supination of the forearm is also possible. To pronate the forearm, it must first be flexed at approximately 90 degrees. Then, rotate your forearm so your palm faces away from your face. To supinate the forearm, rotate it in the opposite direction, bringing the palm towards the face. [31, 36, 37]

4e) Flexion and Extension
Flexion refers to closing a joint or decreasing the angle between two body parts. For example, flexing the arm brings

the forearm so it touches the bicep. Extension of the arm is the opposite motion, increasing the angle between the bicep and the forearm. A flexion of the hip would be a standing forward fold. An extension of the hip would be standing upright or a standing backbend. [31, 30, 38]

4f) Circumduction
Circumduction refers to the rotation of any body part in a circular motion. You trace this motion by picking a point on the body part in motion. The subsequent rotation of that point traces a circle in space. This could be an arm, leg, wrist, ankle, finger, eye, hip, etc. [39]

4g) Medial and Lateral Rotation
Medial rotation refers to the rotation of a limb towards the midline of the body. Begin from a neutral position with the thumb on top. Rotating your thumb counterclockwise will create a medial rotation of the arm. Lateral rotation refers to the rotation of a limb away from the midline of the body. The arm is rotated laterally if the thumb is rotated in a clockwise direction. [31, 40, 41]

4h) Depression and Elevation
Depression and elevation, respectively, refer to the lowering and raising of a body part in a linear motion that is parallel to the centerline of the body. As you raise or lower the body part, the distance between that body part and the centerline of the body is not increased. You might imagine raising or lowering the eyebrows, jaw or shoulders in an elevation or depression. [31,42]

4i) Retraction and Protraction
Retraction and protraction, respectively, mean to move
any body part to the posterior or anterior part of the body.
Imagine what it would look like to retract and protract the
jaw or shoulders.[31,43]

4j) Dorsiflexion and Plantarflexion
Dorsiflexion means to flex the foot bringing the toes up to-
wards the knee. Plantarflexion means to point the toes down
away from the knee. This also pertains to the movement of
the hand. To create a dorsiflexion of the hand extend your
arm so you're looking at the back of your hand and then try
to bring your fingers towards your body. Extend your arm so
your palm faces your body then bring the tips of your fingers
towards your body; this is a plantar flexion of the hand. [31, 44, 45]

4k) Inversion and Eversion
Inversion and eversion, respectively, mean to rotate the foot
(while flat on the floor) towards the midline of the body and
away from the midline of the body.[31, 46]

4l) Geometric
Geometric modifications are standard geometric ways of
animating postures. These modifications include (but are not
limited to) circular, oval, square, arc, linear, twisting, bending
front to back, bending side to side, figure eight, rocking side
to side, and rocking back and forth.

4m) Swapping
Swapping is when you mix part of one pose with part of
another pose. For example you might mix the arm position
from Garuda-asana (eagle pose) with Uttanasana- (stand-
ing forward fold).[1]

Energy/Effort Modifications:

4n) Passive Pose
A passive pose requires little or no effort on the part of the student. An example of this type of pose is shavasana.

4o) Active Pose
An active pose is one that requires effort or muscle energy.

4o1) Active Pose Minimum Effort
Active minimum effort is the minimum effort required to barely hold the pose. This typically results in poor alignment because the student does not have the strength to get the pose to work properly. They may tend to change the shape of the pose to force it to work. For example, in downward dog a student might move their arms so they are more perpendicular to the floor. Students may also lock out joints to accommodate. In all cases the student should be advised to move to a simpler version of the pose that they can do properly. For example, if they cannot hold downward dog you may have them do table or child's.

4o2) Active Pose Activation Effort
Active activation effort refers to exerting the desired amount of effort in order for the pose to work properly. The general concept is that in order to achieve the proper alignment in a pose you must exert a certain amount of effort. This implies a certain amount of strength.

4o3) Active Pose Excess Effort
Active excess effort refers to exerting too much muscle energy. This can result in fatigue, create tension and muscle pulls. This is, in essence, forcing oneself into the posture. The

student has enough strength but not enough flexibility to achieve the posture; by over exerting they force themselves into the shape. This is obviously not a good expression of the posture and is likely to cause injury.

Isometric or Dynamic Poses:

4p1) Isometric Poses
An isometric pose is one like downward dog. Isometric re-fers to the fact that it is fundamentally a stationary pose.[1]

4p2) Dynamic Poses
Dynamic poses are poses that are animated or move in time. An example of this type of pose would be cat cow, during which you actively transition from one pose to the next.[1]

4.1 Establish the Breath and the Core Pose

4.1.1 Before applying any posture modifications, the breath and the core pose should be established.

4.1.2 Whether you set aside a specific time in the beginning of the class to orient your students to the breath, or whether you weave in the breath concepts while you are teaching, some instruction is necessary. While it is beyond the scope of this text to go into any formal breathing techniques, some of the basic metrics and mechanisms of the breath can be found in chapter 2. Understanding these concepts is a useful foundation in guiding the students to a deeper understanding of their breath. Also, some of the material presented in chapter 2 illuminates the purpose of some standard breathing techniques. After the breath has been established, another fundamental technique is to encourage the students to synchronize the breath with movement.[1]

4.1.3 You establish the core pose by instructing the students as to the general alignment of the torso arms, legs, hands, feet, and the head. [1]

This first section is basic and yet is important to mention as a foundation for the material that follows.

4.2 Stretching Modifications

4.2.1 Probably one of the most obvious modifications to a pose is the depth of the stretch. The student has many options here in expressing the pose with a very mild stretch or a stretch at their edge. Depending on how a particular student is feeling, a milder representation of the pose may be exactly what they need. [1]

I would like to set up a metric to help explore this and other ideas presented in the remainder of this chapter. Let's start by defining a scale of 1 to 10, where 10 is your edge (or the deepest stretch that is safe for you) and 1 is barely feeling any stretch at all. Pick different levels within this range and explore what the postures feel like at each.

4.2.2 Next consider how the stretch is distributed through-out the body. Is the stretch concentrated in one small muscle group, or, is it distributed equally throughout the body? In general, the aim of Hatha yoga is to distribute the stretch equally throughout the body, which makes the pose safer and the student less likely to pull or hyperextend a muscle.

This does not mean to use muscles that are not required for the pose.

When the stretch tends to be more concentrated this may mean that a smaller muscle group has a higher degree of tension than the surrounding tissue. This smaller and tighter group of muscles should dictate the degree of stretch.[29]

4.3 Effort or Exertion Modifications

4.3.1 Yoga postures also require effort; the degree of effort available to you is a function of your relative strength in each posture. It is important to be aware of how much effort you are exerting in each posture. If you push too hard you may begin to strain muscles. At any time if a pose begins to strain any muscle group it is best to back out and take a break. See chapter 5 for a deeper explanation of the edge. To the contrary, if you don't push hard enough your body doesn't gain the benefits from the pose. Make sure that the level of effort in each posture is right for you. If you do so you will be building strength and flexibility without causing any harm. Below you will find different classifications of effort.

4.3.2 Passive poses (definition 4n) are poses that require little or no muscle effort. One example of this type of pose is shavasana. There are many poses where the torso is in contact with earth that fall into this category. You may be on your side, back or stomach. Typically, the feet are on the floor; the legs may or may not be in contact with the earth. Also the arms and head are usually in contact with the earth in passive poses.

4.3.3 Active poses require muscle effort (definition 4o). Active poses are all other poses that do not fall into the passive category. As these poses are too numerous to mention I will not try to describe them. Active poses can be isometric or dynamic.

4.3.4 Active Pose Minimum Effort (definition 4o1) is the minimum effort required to barely establish the pose.

Two basic ways active pose minimum effort might manifest:

1) The proper alignment is achieved but for a very short period of time. This implies that the student does not have enough strength to hold the pose in the proper alignment for the specified amount of time. In this case it is advised that the student hold the proper alignment as long as they can and then move out into a more passive pose like table, shavasana, or child's. It is very important for the student to keep the proper alignment even if it is for a very short period of time. Their strength and endurance will increase over time if the pose is practiced in the proper fashion.
2) An improper alignment is achieved. In this case the student has found a way to create the general shape of the pose but with a compromised alignment. It may be that students find this expression because of a lack of strength, motivation, experience, or they are fatigued. In

any case care should be taken not to strain while holding the pose. Sometimes to hold the pose longer they may compensate by further changing the alignment (possibly up to the point where joints are being locked out). This is not recommended.

4.3.5 Active pose activation effort (definition 4o2) is the proper effort (and implied strength level) required to hold a pose with the correct alignment for the prescribed amount of time. This means that you are able to do the pose without straining and are gaining the benefit from the posture. There is a certain feeling of ease in the pose even though you may be exerting significant effort. When this expression of the posture is reached you feel as though you could hold it for a long time.

4.3.6 Active pose excess effort (definition 4o3) refers to exerting too much energy in the pose thus pushing past your edge. This is likely to build tension and be counterproductive. When students exert too much effort they are essentially forcing themselves into the pose. They may be trying to look like the rest of the students in the class no matter how much they have to compromise the alignment and effort.

4.3.7 Next consider how the effort is distributed through the body. Is the majority of the effort concentrated in one small muscle group, or, is it distributed more equally through a larger group of muscles? In general the aim of Hatha yoga to distribute the effort equally throughout as many muscle groups as possible. Distributing the effort through more muscle groups makes the pose safer; you are therefore less likely to pull or hyperextend a muscle. This is also what allows you to hold a pose for longer periods of time. Some poses will inherently focus the effort in smaller or larger muscle groups. Whatever the case may be the aim is to distribute the effort through as many muscle groups as possible. [29]

There are muscles in each pose that are not required. Over time it is the goal of the student to relax these muscles. In other words you don't want to use what you don't need.

4.4 Balance Modifications

4.4.1 Any pose where you are supported by your arms or your legs requires some degree of balancing. The degree varies greatly depending on how supported each pose is. For example, table pose is very supported and doesn't require much balancing. However, tree pose is much less supported and requires much more balancing.

4.4.2 Also consider how the balancing is distributed throughout the body. Standing postures will probably engage the most muscle groups in the act of balancing. Standing balancing poses employ the head, arms, legs, torso, etc. Poses like shavasana, on the other hand, will require no balancing at all. Postures like plank pose require less balancing. Look at each posture that you use and consider which muscle groups are engaged in the act of balancing.

4.4.3 Breath is one of the tools to help the balancing postures. Keeping the breath flowing smoothly and fully is a helpful aid in balancing. If you can modify your breath so that it maintains a full and even character, balancing will most likely be easier for you.[1]

4.4.4 A drishti point is effective in balancing postures. Consider that your concentration may drift away from your drishti. Try to bring your concentration back to that point every time you drift away. [1]

4.4.5 Stressing the core alignment of the spine and legs is important in balancing. Core alignment in the standing poses, addresses the position of the legs and the spine. If you can do the whole pose but have to compromise the core alignment, this is not a good expression. The best solution is to modify the posture so that the core alignment remains uncompromised. When your strength and maturity in the balancing posture progresses so that your core is stable, you can then consider adding the other elements of the pose. [1]

4.4.6 Overcompensation

Overcompensation is when you move too much to com-pensate for being out of balance. For example, let's say you are in tree pose and you begin to fall slightly to the right; the perfect amount of compensation, let's say, is moving one inch to the left. Overcompensating means you move two inches or three inches. What I am trying to suggest here is to minimize your compensation for being out of balance. Try to make very small adjustments to your balance and see if that is of service.

4.5 Spatial Modifications

4.5.1 Spatial modifications deal with the modifications described in definitions 4c through 4m. These describe some of the fundamental ways that each joint of the body can articulate. In order to make these definitions more usable I have tried to generalize where possible. So, if you are looking for ways to modify a pose—whether it be a major or minor modification—you can use these definitions as a guide.

Definition 4l geometric modifications deal with the patterns used in the animation of a posture. For example, while lying on your back and holding your knees into your chest you might consider rocking from side to side or front to back. Sometimes in seated postures instructors animate the torso in a circular or oval shape to stretch the hips and lower back.[1]

Definition 4m swapping, deals with combining pieces of poses. One way to apply this kind of concept would be to mix the arm position from Garuda-asana (Eagle Pose) with Uttanasana- (Standing Forward Fold). There are many other possibilities for swapping. If you are concerned about the combination you are considering consult your physician.[1]

4.6 Duration of any Held Posture

4.6.1 Another way to consider modifying a posture would be its duration or how long it is held. Will you hold the posture for one breath or ten breaths? This section refers to the duration that the pose is held.[1]

4.7 Speed of Movement

4.7.1 Next, consider the speed of the pose or animated series. This is applicable any time you are in motion. Consider how fast you are moving. For example, in a standing side bend, the time that it takes you to move from neutral to the right or left is the speed of the animation. This is a very interesting aspect of animated poses. Notice how your feelings change when you speed up or slow down the animation.[47]

4.8 Animation of One or a Series of Poses

4.8.1 In general, in animated poses or pose series you are always moving except for slight pauses. Some teachers design their whole class this way.

4.8.2 Animating one pose is like slowly moving into the pose from a neutral position; then almost immediately moving back to the neutral position. This pattern is then repeated. You can animate poses at your edge or anywhere below that. This movement, of course, is synchronized with the breath. For instance, in a standing side stretch: first, you begin in the neutral position and then bend to the right. You would pause slightly at your edge and then move back to neutral. You would then do the same thing to the left. You would then repeat this right and left movement for a prescribed number of cycles. An example of animating a series of poses is contained in the classic sun salutation.[1]

4.8.3 The depth of the animation refers to the amplitude of movement. If we consider the side stretch example given above, the movement from neutral to the right or left can be done to your edge or to any fraction of that distance or angle. For example, maybe you find your edge when bending 15 degrees to the left. You might consider warming up this side stretch by only bending 5 or 10 degrees to begin with, then moving to the full 15 after you are warmed up.

4.8.4 Next, consider how the animation is distributed throughout the body. To do this, notice which muscle groups are activated in the animation. For example, there are many more muscle groups activated when animating cobra pose than if you were to just do a simple dorsiflexion of the foot.

4.9 Recursive Poses (or Short Series of Poses)

4.9.1 Recursive poses are poses that are repeated throughout the class for some specific effect. These are different from transitional poses in that transitional poses help to connect and create a smooth flow between two dissimilar poses. A recursive pose is used more for its general calming, relaxing, or rebalancing effect. Recursive poses are different from counter poses in that you can use recursive poses after any pose. Examples of recursive poses are downward dog, child's, shavasana, etc. For example, if you are designing a very strenuous class, you may want to apply child's pose recursively. In other words throughout the whole class you may choose to do three to four strenuous poses then child's.

4.9.2 Recursive small series of poses are a small series of poses used to rebalance out the body. They can be used after many different types of poses. A good example of this is (yeah, you guessed it) the half sun salutation used in Ashtanga classes.

4.10 Posture Modification Concepts Distributed Through the Whole Class

4.10.1 This section deals with distributing the posture modification concepts through the class. The graphs provided below are intended to be used as general guidelines and do not imply an exact science.

4.10.2 Effort distribution will be the first concept dealt with in this section. For example, you may start out with a very gentle effort for warm-up and then gradually build up to about three-quarters of the way through the class then begin to taper off as you move towards shavasana.

To introduce this concept, first picture the duration of the class from start to finish. Next, break the hour class down into ten-minute intervals; then subdivide the effort levels into ten steps. Level 1 effort is a warm-up level; level 10 is at one's edge. So let's say for the first ten minutes we are using level 1 of effort to warm up for students. In the second ten-minute block we will move to a level 3 of effort. In the third ten-minute block we will move to a level 7 of effort. In the fourth ten-minute block we will move to a level 10 of effort. In the fifth ten-minute block we will move to a level 8 of effort. And in the last ten-minute block we will drop down to a level 2 of effort.

In table form it would look like this:

Ten Minute Block	1	2	3	4	5	6
Time Minutes	0 to 10	10 to 20	20 to 30	30 to 40	40 to 50	50 to 60
Effort Level	1	3	7	10	8	2

Table 4.10.1 Effort Levels Distributed Through the Duration of the Class in Table Form

In graph form it would look like this:

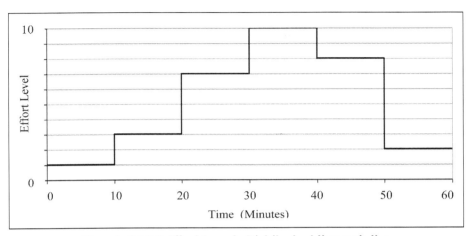

**Graph 4.10.1 Effort Levels Distributed through the
Duration of the Class in Graph Form**

Above is just one example of an effort profile; the possibilities are infinite. Consider that the effort levels can be made smooth. In which case, you could get a graph that looks like the one below. It could actually take on any shape as you desire to benefit your students.

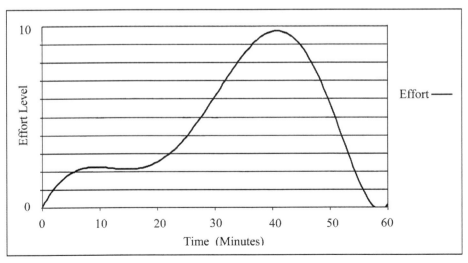

**Graph 4.10.2 Effort Levels Distributed through the Duration
of the Class in Graph Form – Continuous Interpretation**

Continuous interpretation means to smoothen out the profile and make it more gradual as opposed to stepped. You can use whatever form suits your style; both are equally valid.

Note that generating an effort profile in graph form like this is extremely useful. I have created these graphs to help illustrate what they may look like for use in the template described in chapter 7. Understanding the effort profile of your class is a good idea.

4.10.3 You can analyze the stretch distribution profile of your class in much the same way. If we break down the intensity of the stretch from warm-up, which is a level between 0 and 2, and your edge, which is at a level of 8 to 10, we can create the same type of plots for the stretch distribution profile. The possibilities for these profiles are infinitely variable and can take on any shape.

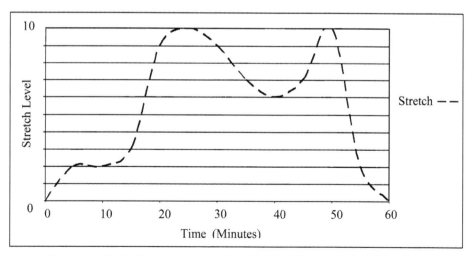

Graph 4.10.3 Stretch Levels Distributed through the Duration of the Class in Graph Form – Continuous Interpretation

4.10.4 The speed of each posture has a strong effect on how the student experiences the posture.

The speed distribution profile of your class can be analyzed in much the same way as stretching or effort. A level 10 is the fastest posture and a level 0 is the slowest. Again remember that speed profiles also can take on any shape. A speed level of 10 would be equivalent to a fast vinyasa class. A speed level of 0 to 1 would be a slow yin class.

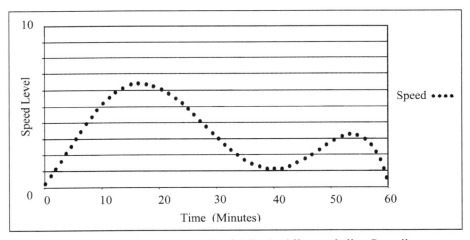

Graph 4.10.4 Speed Levels Distributed through the Duration of the Class in Graph Form — Continuous Interpretation

4.11 Combining Profiles

4.11.1 Let's take a look at the relationship between the pro-files for effort, stretch, and speed (see Fig 4.11.1). In the first fifteen minutes of the class we are at very moderate levels of stretch and effort. However, the speed of the postures during this phase can be moderately high because they are warm-up poses. During normal exercise it is always a good idea to stretch before the effort. This is exactly what is accomplished in the first fifteen to thirty minutes of the class. Also, in that same timeframe we begin to slow more and more and gradually increase the effort. Then, between the thirty- and forty-five-minute phase of class we have the major effort. Note here that the speed is way down for safety but we still have a moderate level of stretch. Then between forty-five and fifty minutes into the class we're increasing the level of stretch again. Here we have designed the effort level to drop off and the speed increases slightly. So what you notice is that we're stretching before and after the major effort of the class. This is a very standard and well accepted practice for many types of physical activity. It is always a good idea to stretch before and after the effort phase of your exercise. Next notice the speed of the execution of these postures. The speed starts out slow but gradually increases to about the fifteen-minute point of the class. Then when the stretching and effort become intense we slow down. At the end of the class, when the stretching and effort taper off, we can increase the speed slightly. In general when doing intense stretching or effort postures it is probably good to slow them down to help protect your students. The warm-up and cool down postures can be done at a greater speed if desired because they are not as demanding or taxing to the body.

The examples given above illustrate only one approach to designing the effort, stretch, and speed levels for a yoga class (the actual possibilities are infinite). Here I have tried to show what a standard type of practice might look like. Just the fact that you can now visualize these variables (as shown in the plots) and see how they relate to one another is a step to deeper understanding. This also gives you more control over specifically designing these parameters into your class.

Now consider other types of relationships:

- Create a class where the effort always stays low but stretch is high
- Maybe design two areas where the effort is high
- Design a vinyasa class where the speed, stretch, and effort are all relatively high

These are just a few examples; the possibilities are infinite.

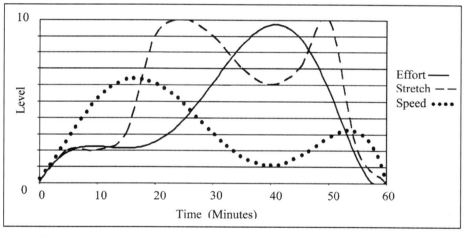

Graph 4.11.1 Combination of Effort Stretch and Speed Profiles throughout the Class in Graph Form —Continuous Interpretation

These tools will enable you to design your own specific intention for your class; but, these levels cannot be rigid. These are only a rough guideline for your teaching style. Every yoga teacher knows that they must be very accommodating to adjust the effort, stretch, and speed levels to suit each class.

Definition 3d from chapter 3 "Test Poses and Other Test Methods," elaborates on some tools that can be used to evaluate the capabilities of your students.

4.12 Use the Concepts in this Chapter to Evaluate Other Teachers' Classes

4.12.1 Note that you can use these tools to analyze other teachers classes; as you are observing notice the distribution of stretch, effort, balance, and speed in their practice. You also may consider the distribution of other elements throughout the class. In general you can use all of the material in this chapter to document and analyze other teachers' classes. Also you can use the class design template shown in chapter 7 to take notes in for the same purpose.

4.13 Use the Concepts of this Chapter to Deeply Investigate any Joint

Two of the books cited in the endnotes "Anatomy of the Human Body" and "Anatomy and Human Movement" are two wonderful companion books for my book. Using the "Anatomy and Human Movement" text you can look up any joint in the body and determine its type and range of motion, muscles used etc. You can then look up the specific muscles and other core anatomy in "Anatomy of the Human Body". Use these to determine what muscles you wish to stretch and what poses will achieve that goal.

❦

5.0 The Edge

5.0.1 In general, we are taught that the edge is the threshold of pain. The concept of straining is also synonymous. It is a state in which you know you shouldn't be. However, we often push into it and sometimes well past it. Anybody who has practiced yoga for more than a few years undoubtedly knows at least a few people who have hurt themselves by going past their edge. When finding the expression of each posture, the edge is definitely one of the limiting factors. [1]

An interesting mechanism within the concept of the edge is what is normally called, "the first edge." This is where you move into a pose and discover the first threshold of pain. Sometimes just pausing there and breathing for a moment the body will open up and allow a deeper expression to a second deeper edge.[1]

There is a subtle distinction that needs to be made here between the threshold of pain and the threshold of fear. If a student is afraid to do a pose this edge needs to be respected in the same manner as if it were physical. This can be very limiting for some students; but yoga in this regard can provide a great potential for growth. When the student is ready they will move.[47]

5.0.2 Most of the time we discuss the physical edge. This normally finds its expression in asking the student to go to the threshold of pain and then back up a little bit. Sometimes the edge manifests itself in the form of holding the breath, typically seen when the physical edge is passed to such a degree that it sends the body into a slight mode of panic. Most teachers will tell you that if you're holding your breath you are probably too deep into the pose. Another common edge within the breath is the rate of breathing. The edge has also been compromised if it is not synchronized with movement. Is the student taking three to four breaths where they are being instructed to take only one? If this occurs, slowing them down or asking them to take a break may be prudent.[1]

The above are the most obvious manifestations of the edge. Below I have listed some of the more subtle. These are more likely to manifest if you have a student who is: recovering from an illness or injury; of advanced age; has some chronic health condition; or is a student with special needs. Students need to know that it is okay to back off when they experience any of these edges. This is what helps keep them safe. It is also incredibly liberating for the students to know this because it gives them permission and the freedom to adjust for whatever their body, mind, or breath should throw at them. Since I've begun studying, I've had several health issues that brought out some of the less common edges; some of the descriptions below are from personal experience.

5.0.3 You've heard that the three most important things in real estate are location, location, location. And I'm sure by analogy that the three most important things in respecting your edge are ego, ego, ego. Being aware of and having control of your ego in relation to your edge is always a very important thing for which to strive. The ego typically gets challenged when the student cannot do the pose as instructed. Teachers who can make their students comfortable with their current abilities will be more successful.

5.0.4 There are some deeper metaphorical meanings embedded in the concept of the edge. One is geared towards encouraging growth through risk. Isn't the concept of the edge synonymous with intelligent risk-taking? For example you're encouraged to adjust the pose till you're just below the threshold of pain. So we are taking a risk in being only a few degrees out of danger. But this is a smart risk; we are testing to see where the danger lies and then moving just inside of that. Just as in real life, we must take risks to grow. Yoga, metaphorically speaking, teaches us how to take risks intelligently.

This is also supported by the concept of being non-competitive. Competition with other students may push a student past their optimal space and cause them harm. Just like the dog who has a bone: seeing his reflection in the water he tries to take the bone away from the other dog and loses his own. When competing during yoga we run the risk of losing what we have worked so hard to attain and build. Injuries can sometimes take years to heal and can also be very expensive. Is it really worth the risk? Explaining this to students from this perspective may prove to be beneficial.

5.1 The Edge as Manifested in Muscle Tissue

5.1.1 Muscle or Connective Tissue Pain

Muscle or connective tissue pain (straining) is one of the major expressions of the edge. This is most likely responsible for the feeling of pain experienced when slightly past the edge. Moving deeper into the pose while in this state increases the risk of injury. It is up to the student at this point to back out of the pose somewhat so as not to cause any damage.

5.1.2 Hyperextension with No Immediate Pain

There are muscle and connective tissue groups in the body that are very strong and can handle a great deal of tension with no pain. This does not mean that it is acceptable to bring these muscles into that state. This is still past the edge.

Let's take a seated forward fold for example. I am a runner and runners typically have a lot of tension in their legs. Very early in my yoga studies I can remember pushing myself very deeply, forcing myself to grab my feet. My thigh and calf muscles were extremely tight and I could feel that. However, they did not hurt so I stayed in the pose. The next day I found myself suffering from hyperextensions in both my knees and ankles and could barely walk. This injury took months to heal and was totally my fault. I learned the importance of this edge here. The penalty for passing this edge was severe.

5.1.3 Muscle Pull

In this type of injury it is evident immediately that something is wrong. There is an sensation of pain in the muscle tissue.

5.1.4 General strength

Sometimes certain muscle groups may not have the strength to do a pose properly. In these cases it is important to modify the pose so the student can do it comfortably.

5.1.5 Fatigue

When energy runs low, we experience fatigue. Students may only have the strength to do a particular pose properly for a short period of time. Instruct the student to do the pose for as long as they can do it correctly.

5.1.6 Muscle Panic

Students may have the flexibility to go deeper into a pose. However, when muscles are pushed past their typical range of motion there is sometimes an emotional reaction; the muscle will tighten up to protect itself. They may also experience this when doing a pose that they have never done before. Simply relaxing and breathing will sometimes allow the student to move deeper into a pose.

5.1.7 Muscle cramps

Muscle cramps or muscle spasms are involuntarily contractions in the muscle.

5.1.8 Balance

One common edge in balancing (in standing postures) is the straining experienced when struggling too hard. It typically looks like quick movements from side to side (or other directions) to try to steady the pose. The location of this straining is typically in the foot ankle and calf muscles. This can sometimes be accompanied by a great deal of tension in the same areas. It may be best to adjust or exit the pose if this occurs as sustaining this struggle typically builds tension.

5.1.9 Slightly Strained or Tight Muscle

In general, a very tight or slightly strained muscle may not be open to being stretched. If attempted, it may react by tightening up. One approach is to avoid stretching the injured or tight muscle at all. Only stretch the muscles around it. Or you can see if the tender muscle can withstand a gentle stretch. If there is no associated pain it is probably okay.

I have experienced a tight muscle relaxing during a one-hour yoga session by only stretching the muscles around it. It did take a great deal of concentration.

5.1.10 Actual Muscle Strain or Pull

If this condition is present, the essence of healing will reside strongly in the ego. Putting the ego aside and being patient is so important because the muscle or connective tissue needs to be left alone to heal. It can sometimes take months or even years for a serious pull to heal.

I have experienced this personally; while playing soccer, I severely pulled both of my psoas muscles. It took three years for them to heal completely. After four years I am just getting rid of the residual tension. Soon after the pull occurred I went back to practicing yoga and pushed myself too hard. I am certain that the three-year healing process would have been shorter had I backed off more. I stayed with my Ashtanga practice because the muscles were actively healing. However, because I was still taxing them, after about six months the healing stopped. Therefore, I gave up Ashtanga for about a year and a half. That allowed them to continue to heal. Massage therapy was particularly helpful in getting the muscles to let go and allow them to finally heal completely.

5.1.11 Chronic Injuries

For those of us who have chronic injuries getting control of the ego and practicing extreme patience is not a weekly or monthly endeavor. In this case it needs to become a lifetime practice. There is a special concern in chronic injuries especially when the injury is asymmetrical. The concern here is stretching one side of the body more than the other. This occurs because the side that is less injured is often more flexible. If it is continually stretched deeper than the injured side it may continually open up more. Over a great deal of time this is likely to exacerbate the asymmetry. It is wise to keep this in mind and always strive for a sense of balance on each side. In these matters it is important to seek the advice of your doctor prior to doing any yoga practice.

5.2 Edges Expressed in Other Systems of the Body

5.2.1 Breath Holding and Rapid Breathing

Breath holding is a sign that an edge has been passed. Since it is one of the more common symptoms it can be easily identified and corrected. Rapid breathing is another common edge and may be a sign that fatigue is setting in. In either case encourage the student to adjust by backing out or taking a break.

5.2.2 Emotional Edges

Emotional edges exist also; the one I would like to address here is fear. Moving the body in a manner or to a depth that has not experienced before can sometimes induce fear. They may have the ability to go into the pose but they just don't want to. The reasons are not important. What is important is that they respect the discomfort and back out when uncomfortable. [47]

Students in this situation have great potential for growth. Understanding that the limitation is partly emotional is a big step. The next thing is to work with this edge in the same manner as a physical edge. Stay just inside of it, breathe, and when ready, the fear may pass and the pose may open.

5.2.3 Visceral Edge

The visceral edge may manifest in gastrointestinal discomfort and or abdominal tension. In extreme cases it may elevate to feeling nauseous. One possible way to alleviate this is to leave several hours between a meal and your yoga practice. However, there are other things that can bring you to this edge.

One small caveat for me is that I have low blood sugar and find it beneficial to eat a small snack immediately before a yoga practice. I cannot make it through a practice without my sugar running dangerously low. I have found that a small meal of some vegetables, cheese, and bread are ideal for me and have never given me any visceral issues.

5.2.4 Thermal Edge

In general students should not be too warm or too cold in a practice. Elevated temperatures can cause dehydration. There are yoga styles such as Ashtanga and Bikram that are done at elevated temperatures. To keep your body from losing too much water, it is important to be properly hydrated before class.

5.2.5 Blood Sugar

If you start a yoga class with lower blood sugar levels they may drop even lower due to the physical exertion. Eating wisely is important. If you are having issues with blood sugar you may want to contact your doctor or nutritionist.

5.2.6 Heart Rate

Sometimes during a yoga class involving much physical exertion a student may experience an elevated heart rate. To understand a healthy heart rate for your age and health contact your physician. I have noticed that sometimes when tired, isometric poses have caused my heart rate increase rapidly. Please be kind to yourself and back out of the pose if you experience this.

5.2.7 Blood Pressure

Consult with your physician prior to doing a yoga practice if you have blood pressure issues. Also, be sure to disclose the type of class and the level of effort involved.

5.2.8 Concentration Drift

In any yoga pose, it is optimal to maintain concentration on the breath and sensations within the pose. However, it is very difficult to achieve this. It is common to have other thoughts arise. Continue to move the students back to the focal points that you as a teacher find important. Concentration has an edge in this manner so let the students know that it is normal to have it vary. In time when they are ready their concentration will improve and they will find a deeper mental state with fewer interruptive thoughts. [1]

Another area where concentration drift is particularly important is in relation to balancing poses. There is more going on in balancing poses than in most other postures so concentration is further challenged.

You may want to caution your class about concentration drift when doing any pose that requires fine motor skills. This is especially important if the pose has considerable effort involved or if there is some risk of falling out of the pose.

5.2.9 Visual

One of the first tests of the edge is to sit quietly with eyes closed. For those who have a lot of mental activity this may be a significant challenge. When working with a group of people, one of the ways to find out how comfortable they are with sitting quietly is to ask them to sit with their eyes closed. Look around the room as the students attempt to do this exercise. You may find that some will open their eyes or may have trouble sitting still. Be sensitive to this and allow them an out if needed.

5.2.10 Any Other System Unbalance Or Challenge

In general, if any other system in the body becomes over-loaded during yoga it is also an expression of the edge. I have listed some in sections 5.3 through 5.9. You may also find issues with blurred vision, old injuries, nerve pain, or other systems in the body. Take care to honor all of these and let your students know they can back out when necessary.

5.3 Edge Modification Concepts

5.3.1 Ego-Challenging Exercise

Here is an exercise to help students become more com-fortable in respecting their edge: Have one student assume that they are injured and much less flexible than normal. Have them execute the pose only half way to their edge, then look around the room at other students experiencing a much deeper expression of the pose. This is what it might feel like if they were injured.

5.3.2 Dynamic Edge

Typically, as students enter a pose they reach the first edge. They should stop there and back up a little. The next step is to be patient, breathe, and relax. Sometimes the body will open up and allow movement past this first edge into a deeper state of the pose. [1]

5.3.3 Your Edge Changes over Time

All teachers know that during longer term yoga practice the body will more permanently open, thus redefining the edge. For example, after a year or so of practicing yoga the body may be able to stretch deeper in certain poses. Your range of motion has increased in those poses.

Don't feel discouraged if you should become less flexible at times. This will happen in the normal course of development. It can sometimes be brought on by injury, cold temperatures, advancing age, inactivity, or overexertion during uncommon activities.

5.3.4 Heightened Awareness

One of yoga's general purposes is to create a greater sense of inner awareness of the body and mind. If one can come about in this development in the normal course of practice, great. However, some people learn this greater inner awareness only after they have been injured (there are some very interesting stories on this topic). The reason for this is to protect the injured muscles, ligaments, or tendons, extreme care and mindfulness is required. That injured muscle forces students to achieve a greater sense of awareness. In time it should heal, but if students try to stretch the injured muscle they may do more damage. This is from where the motivation comes.

5.3.5 Playing the Edge and Release

While at the edge, students can find greater release by using slight modifications to alignment. This of course will be different for each individual but is important to explore and is one of the finer points of a yoga practice. The teacher can describe the majority of the alignment issues for the pose, but the last small percentage is up to the student. The student will need to explore and test the subtle expressions of alignment in order to find a greater release (refer to chapter 4 for posture modification concepts). This may be explored by adjusting the pose angles, the depth of stretch, the amount of effort, the speed, focus, and breath awareness. [29]

5.3.6 Work Distribution

Another general concept of the edge is finding a way to distribute the work over as many muscles as possible. For example, if in a pose and 90 percent of the work is in one muscle or small group of muscles the pose alignment may be wrong. With this expression of a posture quick fatigue is likely. The body may also be close to injury. The idea is to distribute the load over as many muscle groups as possible. As a student achieves this the poses should move to a sense of effortlessness. This will allow them to hold the pose for much longer, which is one of the fundamental goals of a yoga practice. [29]

To the contrary there are muscle groups that are not required in a pose. This does not mean to use those unnecessary muscles. Any muscle groups that are not required should remain relaxed.

5.3.7 Animated Vs. Stationary Poses

In general one should be aware that animating a pose tends to make it easier. Poses held stationary for longer periods (Yin yoga) of time will be more difficult. [1]

5.3.8 Edge and Temperature

As the temperature in the room increases students should become more flexible. Having a healthy awareness of this and a respect for how your students' bodies change with temperature will benefit the class. When the humidity of the room increases it is harder for the body to cool itself with evaporative cooling, therefore the body will tend to be warmer.

5.3.9 Attitude

Often times it is heard, "I'm just not flexible enough to do yoga." What this normally means is, "My poses don't look as good nor are they as deep as the other students in the class." This is sad and a huge waste if it discourages a student. If a student maintains a deep respect for the edge, many body types in many different states of health state can do yoga safely. Yoga has very little to do with each student's relative flexibility. Everybody has a different physiology that will define how their body moves, where their edge is, and the pace at which their body will open up.

This is where the honor resides in respecting ability. With an enlightened attitude each student can shine in whatever their body lends on any given day. This is something to be proud of.

5.3.10 The Edge as a Litmus Test

You're probably thinking, "Well, there's a strange sounding concept if I ever heard one," but bear with me for a moment. What I mean is to use the edge as a tool to find aches and pains and then try to discover their source. After finding the source you may be able to remove the source of the problem and thus remove the pain.

Yoga is a great tool with which to discover all your little aches and pains because over time it tends to stretch many if not all of the muscles in your body. So if there is a problem somewhere you will normally find it. Let's say your right hand always tends to hurt when you do downward dog. The first thing to do is to pay very close attention to the exact location of the pain. The next thing to do is to keep that location in mind throughout your day. You may find that that exact location hurts badly whenever you are unscrewing a stuck jar lid. This may mean that performing this activity is the cause of the pain in that location. Try to find some other way of opening the lid. Maybe you purchase one of those tools with a handle to give you better leverage. Try this for a week or so and then pay close attention in your yoga practice. You may be surprised to find out that your right hand no longer hurts during downward dog.

This was the case for me. While observing my daily routine I found that while squeezing the plastic bottle of my contact lens solution my right hand hurt in the exact location I had problems in downward dog. So I started using my left hand to squeeze the bottle. I did this for a week or so and the pain went away while in dog. Now I alternate hands to alleviate this pain.

I also found at one point that my knees were aching in poses like janu shirasana and heroes pose. I observed my daily routine for activity that tended to irritate my knees. Then I found it: it was my morning meditation in heroes pose. To remedy this I built myself a small stool to elevate my hips and decrease the tension in my knees. After doing my morning meditation with the stool for about three to four weeks I noticed that I no longer had any pain in my knees during my yoga practice.

It is also possible that the primary activity that is causing the muscles to be overstressed (heaven forbid) is another yoga pose.

What we find here is that the edge can be used as a tool to find issues of localized pain during your yoga practice. By keeping that location in mind during your daily routine (and yoga practice) you may find the source activity that is overloading that area. You discover this by noticing what activity in your daily routine (or yoga practice) that tends to irritate the exact same location. Once you have identified this activity you can try alternative activities that do not irritate that location. You'll need to carry out these alternate activities for a period of time in order for them to be successful. Then pay close attention in your next yoga practice to see if the pain has gone away. If it has, seek to make these changes permanent.

5.3.11 Yoga Off the Mat

I have taught yoga in community settings where some people are not even comfortable getting on a mat. This is important in that their edge is so strong that they cannot even bear to do the poses. What this means to me is that their expression of yoga is just watching. For now that is all they are capable of doing. This is important to respect. Maybe in time they will open up and try it, but for now this is all they are capable of.

5.3.12 One Possible Metaphoric Meaning of the Edge

The edge has a metaphoric psychological meaning as well as the ones described above. Those who are actively working on their edge (for a long period of time) in a physical sense may unconsciously transfer this mechanism to their intellectual and psychological growth as well. The metaphor would specifically manifest as expressing yourself to a fuller extent of who you are both personally and intellectually. The process of opening would be similar to the physical. This is like finding your edge of discomfort of your personality and intellect. Then you do your personal and intellectual work just inside their thresholds of pain. Working in this state is like taking healthy risks. Compare this to breathing and relaxing once you have found your first edge to see if, in simply relaxing, you can exceed it. Learning how to take intelligent risks in order to grow is the idea in both cases.

In yoga communities the goal is to accept a person's abilities and person without challenge. Who they are and their talents are not compared to others, judged, or criticized. Think about it: you are encouraged to go to the extent of your abilities (your edge) and then challenge yourself there. The practice of yoga, therefore, encourages you to an enlightened meaning of personal and intellectual (and physical of course) growth. This is to challenge yourself, at your level of ability and your own pace. I believe that the fathers of yoga, with incredible wisdom and insight, designed these concepts in order to optimize the growth of each student. It is also a concept of healing and self compassion on the part of the student. This is where each personal light shines, grows, and flourishes.

Let's take this argument one step further and look at the sum total of all of the possible edges that exist for us in this human form. If we can come to total acceptance of each and every one of them (or total acceptance of yourself) and work patiently only taking intelligent risks, we might find a very beautiful expression of life. The potential for beauty, serenity, healing, and growth is accelerated in this state of mind.

This is one of the deepest expressions of health and beauty that I have ever experienced.

First, you are challenged to be exactly who you are with none of the social, political, or peer pressure masks. Then you are encouraged to exceed that. You are asked to do this consistently over time and grow (by pushing your edge) deeper into the person that you need to be.

✿

6.0 Special Needs

6.1 General Comments

6.1.1 The easiest way to communicate the concept of the edge to your class is to tell them that, "Nothing should hurt." This is the simplest expression of the edge and it communicates very well to a very large cross section of people. [48]

6.1.2 Most people do not have much trouble in a yoga class but when considering people with physical or emotional issues, pregnant women, those who are overweight, etc., consider that all of the edges in chapter 5 become more important. We will certainly find that a greater percentage of these edges will manifest in special-needs groups. Try to determine which of these edges are most likely to manifest in the group with which you are working and develop strategies to protect your class.

6.1.3 Use the test pose techniques described in definition 3d to help determine the general edge of your class.

6.1.4 When dealing with people with special needs, avoid putting them in poses that require fine motor skills. This means you don't want to create a situation where a small compromise in strength, concentration or balance will cause the student to fall out of the pose. Poses to avoid in this case are shoulder stand, headstand, wheel pose, etc.

7.0 Definition of the Class Design Template "Pulling it all Together"

7.0.1 Before or after reading this chapter you can read box 0.3 in the introduction for another explanation on how this box works.

You may now wish to gather some of your favorite posture references. It may serve you to refer to them to create some initial ideas while reading this chapter. You may wish to make some initial attempts to fill in the template as you read along.

7.0.2 Overview of Chapter 7 and the Class Design Template

Chapter 7 is strictly a set of definitions for each box or series of boxes and gives you an idea on how to fill them in.

In chapters 1 through 6 many components of yoga Class Design have been presented. Once you have decided on what type of class you wish to design, the template provides guidance on selecting and organizing that information into a class.

Let's proceed by reviewing the actual image of the template as shown in figure 7.1.1. You'll see a series of boxes with letters and numbers in the upper left-hand corner. The letters are there for reference only. For example, the first box in the upper left-hand corner is labeled "a." Definition 7a (shown below) is the definition on how that box is filled in or used. The numbers 1 through 48 in box "o" are used to sketch or name the postures you will use. So, if you wanted to refer to a posture, you could do so by calling it posture fifteen or twenty, etc. The words in some of the boxes provide guidance on how to fill in or use that box. Box "g" has a capital "P" below it. This "P" stands for progression (definition 3l) or the order of the pose categories (definition 3k) throughout the class. One example of a pose progression might be standing, seated, inversions, on back, on stomach, etc.

Figure 7.1.2 presents an overview of the template in a different way. For clarity I try to present the important concepts in this book in three or four different ways. Take a moment to review this figure as I take us through the steps in using the template in more detail. Note that each callout box has a step number in the upper left-hand corner in bold. Following the step numbers in numerical order is the general way to use the template.

Figure 7.1.3 describes in more detail the relationship between the effort, stretch, and speed curves, the pose progression in column g, and the actual postures sketched in box o. Also refer to Figure 0.2 for further explanation.

The template can be used to design a class of any length.

7.0.3 Some Benefits Gained by Using the Template

The template serves to preserve the ideas and build / revise to constantly improve your teaching skills. For example, if you have a detailed document of each one of your class types, this serves as a preserving foundation and easily allows you to build upon it. Continually consolidate your ideas onto one template for any particular class type. Over the years this will bring a wealth of knowledge together to continually raise your level of teaching. As we progress through our careers it is easy to forget some of our past successful teaching styles and class posture content. This template will give you a medium to not only preserve but also to build upon them.

Every time you get a new idea for a class, create a quick sketch of it in the template. Even if it is just a skeletal outline of the class, it will serve to preserve your idea. Ideas are often fleeting and sometimes lost when not documented.

For example, if you tend to like to free associate your class you may just want to put down rough ideas into your class design template. You can use this as a frame work to free associate on. On the other hand, if you like to go into great detail into the specifics of creating a yoga class, this template will serve that purpose also. I give several methods in chapter 8 on how to design a class in a very intentional manner for a specific purpose.

This is an outstanding tool for teaching and conveying preconceived ideas to other teachers. It provides a standard template in which to share class design ideas: formal training, seminars, or casual sharing of ideas.

Students in formal yoga training, attending seminars, observing another teacher's class, or in any other type of learning environment can use the template to take notes. The template provides excellent reminders for the major facets of the class. It will key the observer's mind in to these elements and provide them a space (and nomenclature) for documentation of these elements. Once recorded in this fashion the notes are immediately organized for easy future reference. This is a very good way to preserve the meaning of the notes you are taking. When you go back to notes taken in this manner over a long period of time you will be able to make much more sense of them.

Using this text and template there are an unlimited number of ways to create and modify a class or program (series of classes).

7.1 Definitions of the Boxes in the Template

The lettered definitions below refer to the boxes with the same letter in the class design template (see Fig 7.1.1 and 7.1.2). For example definition 7a refers to box "a" in the template. This chapter defines what the author can enter into each of the boxes to create their class. Of course, remember that this is designed to be flexible so experiment and come up with your own novel approaches / use. In other words, this is far from an exact science so you can use these techniques as described in this text in any part or whole. The exciting thing is that you can create your own derivative methods from this text. Once you have the format and syntax the possibilities are endless. For now, let's come back to the basics and define the class design template.

7a) Box "a": Major Subject of the Class
Select the major subject of the class. For example, do you wish to create a general purpose class, a class for the back, an aggressive vinyasa flow, etc.?

This book gives some general guidelines in chapter 3 for these decisions.

7b) Box "b": Class Author and Class Type
1) The author
2) The date that the class was designed
3) Place a check in front of the program text if you are defining a program
4) If it is a program that you are defining enter the number of this class out of the total number of classes. It would look something like: 1of 5, 3 of 4, etc.
5) Place a check in front of the single class text you are only creating a single class.

7c) Box "c": Class References
This box gives you a space to include the references that you used to create this class. For example what books, magazine articles, or personal notes did you use?

7d) Box "d" Class Preparation
In box "d" enter ideas on how you would like to prepare the class. Depending on what type of class you will be conducting you will set it up differently and use different props or aids. In this box you'll generally enter your desires on:

preparing the room lighting and temperature, how you would like to arrange the students, what type of props you might need like blankets straps or blocks, what types of CDs to use for background music, including incense or aromatherapy oils, and any other preparation ideas you might have.

Chapter 1, sections 1.1 through 1.3.4 give some guidelines on class preparation.

7e) Box "e": Opening Dialogue
Box "e" provides a space to enter your main ideas on your opening dialogue. The opening dialogue should generally prepare the students for the type of class you will teach. It should introduce them to your main intention and give them some idea about how they will carry that out. This box might also include: an introduction of the edge, inquiring about injured students, letting go of daily issues, moving students to an inward focus, presenting some ideas about the breath and maybe some intention on creating a sacred space.

Chapter 1, sections 1.4.1 through 1.4.7 give guidelines on how to create the opening dialog.

7f) Box "f": Recurrent Themes
Box "f" is a space for you to enter the recurrent themes that you would like to periodically introduce to your students throughout the class. Letting go of your daily concerns, allowing thoughts to arise and pass, the breath, and the edge are all examples of things you might bring up recursively during the class. This box can also be used to list the things of which you want to remind yourself while teaching.

Chapter 1, sections 1.5.1 and 1.5.2 give guidelines on recurrent themes for the students and you.

7g) Box "g" (column): Pose Categories and Progressions (definitions 3k and 3l)
Box "g" is reserved for the categories and progressions. This is where you dictate the pose categories (definition 3k) that you will execute. For example, you may begin with a group of seated poses followed by a group of the back, on the stomach, inversions, and so on. There are progressions like these listed in yoga textbooks.

Chapter 3 section 3.3.4 gives some ideas about creating a progression for your class.

7h) Item "h" (curve): Effort Modifications (shown as a solid line in the template)
Effort modifications are defined by sketching a curve that represents the effort level that will be used for each group of postures. This curve defines the effort level throughout the class. For example you want to begin every class at a lower effort level so the students can warm up gradually. Then you could increase the effort gradually to a maximum level and then taper it off slowly towards the end of the class. Note that all curves are sketched in the same large rectangular box as shown in figure 8.1.1.

Chapter 4 section 4.10.2 describes the concept of effort modifications throughout the class. Sketch this curve appropriately into the box provided. You are not copying what I have provided; the idea here is to create your own effort curve. Remember that the lower values are to the left in the box and the higher are to the right. This concept holds

*true for all curves sketched in that box. For further explana-
tion you can refer to step 8 in figure 7.1.2. Also, table 4.10.1
and graphs 4.10.1 and 4.10.2 describe this concept. (Table
4.10.1 and graph 4.10.1 are really introductory concepts;
the final intent for application is graph 4.10.2.)*

*7i) Item "i" (curve): Stretch Modifications (shown as a dashed
line)*
*Stretch modifications are defined by sketching a curve
that represents the stretch level that you wish to use for
each group of postures. This curve defines the stretch
level throughout the whole class. For example you may
wish to start out with mild stretches in the beginning of the
class so the students can warm up slowly. Then gradually
increase the depth of the stretch and finally we will taper
it off towards the end of class. For further explanation you
can refer to step 8 in figure 7.1.2.*

*Chapter 4 section 4.10.3 describes the concept of stretch
modifications throughout the class. Graph 4.10.3 helps describe this concept in graph form.*

*7j) Item "j" (curve): Speed Modifications (shown as a dotted
line)*
*Speed modifications are defined by sketching a curve that
represents the level of speed at which you want each group
of postures to proceed. This curve defines the speed level of
the postures throughout the whole class. For example if you
are going to design a yin yoga class the speed would be
very slow throughout. To the contrary if you are going to design a vinyasa class speed will be greater, possibly towards
the maximum. For further explanation you can refer to step
8 in figure 7.1.2.*

Chapter 4 section 4.10.4 describes the concept of speed modifications throughout the class. Graph 4.10.4 helps describe this concept.

The relationships between curves "h," "i," and "j" are described in chapter 4.11 and graph 4.11.1. These will help you fine tune the curves to get the desired effect for your class.

Note that you can also include any other concepts in this section. You may come up with other metrics that you would like to track throughout the class. Use this section to plot out the intensity of your own metrics throughout your class. For example, you may wish to track the depth of breath that you present to your students or the degree of balance.

7k) Item "k": Major Pose Expansion Technique
Note:
The box including letters "k," " l," and "m" are concerned with the organization, modification, and development of the poses sketched or named in section "o," which refers to boxes 1 through 48. No data is actually entered for sections "k," "l" and "m;" they are only there for your reference on ideas for filling in the boxes in section "o."

Chapter 3 definitions 3c, 3e, 3f, and 3g describe a classical way of expanding on a major pose (or poses) to create a small flow or your whole class. This basically entails selecting a major pose, then providing an introductory pose to be used before it. After the major pose, insert a counter pose, then lastly a transitional pose that flows naturally between the last counter pose and the next introductory pose.

Also refer to sections 3.3.2 through 3.3.3 for more of an explanation.

7l) Item "l": Pose Flow Development
Pose flow development refers to how the poses relate to one another. For example you may wish to have a series of smoothly flowing postures. You could also develop a flow that is intentional on how each pose relates to the last one as far as the benefits to the body, mind, or some other aspect.

See chapter 3 definitions 3m through 3u. Chapter 3 gives some core tools on how to create the flow of poses for your class.

7m) Item "m": Pose Modification Concepts
Once the breath and the core pose have been established you may choose to modify the pose in some way. For example, you may begin tree pose with the hands in prayer at the heart. You might then modify it by bringing the hands out to the side and then over the head.

See chapter 4 all definitions. Chapter 4 gives many suggestions on how to modify a pose once you have established it.

7n) Item " n" (column): Other Pose Modification Concepts and General Notes
Section "n" is the column of blank boxes that run the length of the template. These spaces are for including notes relative to the poses listed in the same row. Or you can use these cells for any types of notes that you would like to include.

In general you may include posture modification concepts, specific breathing instructions, how many times to repeat a sequence of postures, etc.

7o) Boxes "o" (1-48): Pose Sketches and or Pose Names
Boxes marked "o" define the series of rectangles numbered 1 through 48. The purpose for it is to sketch a stick figure pose or write the names of the poses that you will use in your class. See step 10 in figure 7.1.2 for more instructions. Definitions 3m through 3u give some suggestions on how to create your progressions.

7p) Box "p": Shavasana and Closing Notes
Box "p" is for comments on shavasana. For example you may have some special notes on how to transition your class into shivasana. You can also include how to awaken your class. You also may wish to put in some comments on how to close the class.

Refer to figure 7.1.2 for a concise summary of what we just covered. This is your quick reference guide (cheat sheet). If you are using the guide and have more questions you can always refer back to the definitions in section 7.1.

a) Major Subject & Purpose:	b) Author: Date: / / Program : Class: of Single Class:		c)References:
d) Preparation:	e) Opening Dialogue:		f) Recurrent Themes:

g) P	h) Effort — i) Stretch - - - j) Speed • • • •	*(min)* *(max)*	k) See definitions 3c to 3j for basic pose classifications l) See definitions 3m to 3u for pose series concepts m) See chapter 4 posture modification concepts			n) Notes:
			o)1	2	3	4
			5	6	7	8
			9	10	11	12
			13	14	15	16
			17	18	19	20
			21	22	23	24
			25	26	27	28
			29	30	31	32
			33	34	35	36
			37	38	39	40
			41	42	43	44
			45	46	47	48
p) Shavasana / Awakening From Shavasana / Closing Dialogue:						

Table 7.1.1 Yoga Class Blank Design Template   (by: David Trimboli)

Step 1 Box "a" is for the major subject and purpose

Step 2 Box "b" is for general info

Step 5 Box "e" is for opening dialogue

Step 3 Box "c" is for references used

Step 4 Box "d" is for class preparation items

Step 6 Box "f" is for recurrent themes

Step 7 The boxes in column "g" are for pose categories like: standing, sitting, inversions etc. Each box generally refers to its adjacent row.

If the first box in section "g" read "sitting" then the boxes marked 1, 2, 3, and 4 in section "o" would generally be seated postures.

This is only a general rule. If there are other types of poses in boxes 1 through 4 that's ok.

Step 9 Box 9 gives ways to manipulate section "o". See Table 7.1.1 for actual text

Step 11 The boxes in column "n" are for any other notes

Step 12 Fill in box "p" with instructions to enter shavasana, how to awaken from shavasana and any closing comments

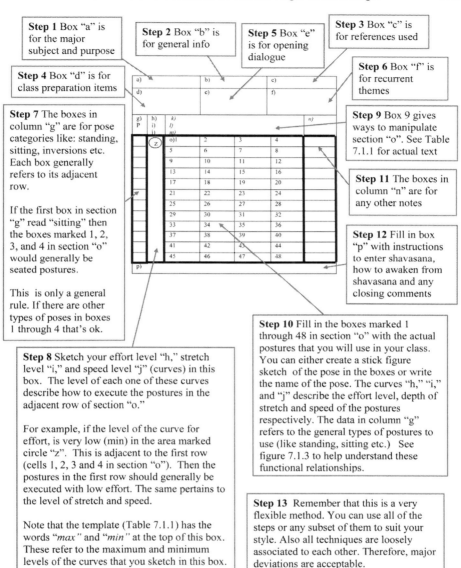

Step 8 Sketch your effort level "h," stretch level "i," and speed level "j" (curves) in this box. The level of each one of these curves describe how to execute the postures in the adjacent row of section "o."

For example, if the level of the curve for effort, is very low (min) in the area marked circle "z". This is adjacent to the first row (cells 1, 2, 3 and 4 in section "o"). Then the postures in the first row should generally be executed with low effort. The same pertains to the level of stretch and speed.

Note that the template (Table 7.1.1) has the words "*max*" and "*min*" at the top of this box. These refer to the maximum and minimum levels of the curves that you sketch in this box.

Step 10 Fill in the boxes marked 1 through 48 in section "o" with the actual postures that you will use in your class. You can either create a stick figure sketch of the pose in the boxes or write the name of the pose. The curves "h," "i," and "j" describe the effort level, depth of stretch and speed of the postures respectively. The data in column "g" refers to the general types of postures to use (like standing, sitting etc.) See figure 7.1.3 to help understand these functional relationships.

Step 13 Remember that this is a very flexible method. You can use all of the steps or any subset of them to suit your style. Also all techniques are loosely associated to each other. Therefore, major deviations are acceptable.

Figure 7.1.2 Schematic of Template and Definitions Showing General Steps

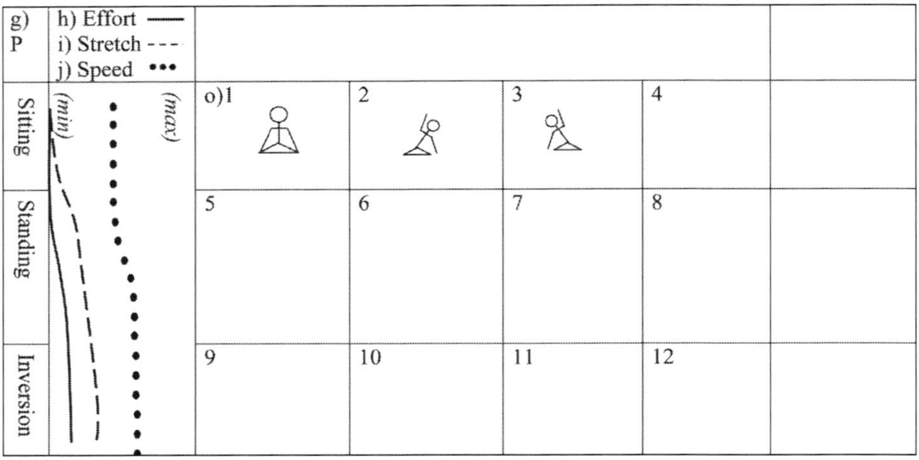

g) P	h) Effort ——— i) Stretch - - - j) Speed •••					
Sitting	(min) • (max)	o)1	2	3	4	
Standing		5	6	7	8	
Inversion		9	10	11	12	

Figure 7.1.3 Understanding The Relationship between Section "g," Curves "h," "i" and "j" and Section "o"

The first row of postures (boxes 1, 2, 3, and 4) should generally be sitting poses by your design because the box in section g of the same row says sitting. Likewise, the postures in the 2nd row (boxes 5, 6, 7, and 8) should in general be standing postures.

Continuing, the curves that you designed for effort "h," stretch level "i," and speed "j" are also designed to impact the choice of postures in section "o". For example, note that the solid line "h" is at the minimum in the first row, meaning that you want to choose postures for that row that have very little effort. The curve for stretch is very low but is ramping up, which means that you will start with a very mild stretch and gradually increase it. And the postures will proceed at an average speed half way between the maximum (fast vinyasa) and minimum (yin yoga or restorative speed). Continue to form these relationships for the remainder of the rows in your template. Use only the number of rows required to suit your class duration / subject and purpose.

The guidelines described above for column "g" and curves "h," "i" and "j" are only general guidelines; remember, this is not an exact science.

See also Fig 0.2 in the introduction and the associated text below it.

For a completed example see figure 8.1.1.

Phew! That was a lot of conceptual information. You should now have a pretty good idea of how this system works. You may find that you are now asking yourself, "How will I find a method that works for me?" Don't fret: that is exactly what the last chapter is designed to do.

Chapter 8 gives you twenty-three graduated methods of using the template. Each method is an easy-to-follow, step-by-step procedure. The beginning methods are very simple and they gradually build in difficulty. Each method attempts to focus on class design from a different perspective. Working through these exercises will build on your expertise in yoga class design. As in any discipline, the more variation you use in the creation of your product the deeper you will understand it and the greater control you will leverage over it.

As you work through the exercises in chapter 8 try to search out which ones work best for you.

❧

8.0 Using and Applying the Class Design Template

Now that we have defined a wealth of facets for yoga class design and defined a template to organize and develop them the next task is to define some methods of using the template.

Once you find a few that you like, I would like to encourage you to continually push yourself and try some methods below with which you are not comfortable. Even if it is only an academic exercise it may serve you to work through some of the other methods presented. The benefit of this is that you learn your craft more thoroughly. Approaching any discipline from many different perspectives can only add to your ability to create a class on a higher level. Some of these methods are only incrementally different from each other and some are vastly different.

You may find it useful to have your favorite posture sources and other reference information available while working through the exercises in this chapter.

As a reminder, I sometimes use the word "component(s)" to refer to the material presented in chapters 1 through 6. This could refer to the whole body of that information any subset or any single item.

As you work through these exercises pay attention to how much of your own unique voice and creativity become part of your class. These exercises will actively engage you in a high-level creative process.

Section 8.3.1 is a special milestone in this process. Reaching it will allow you to leverage the sum total of the information in this text. It also creates reminders and insertion points for information that you already have.

When you get to section 8.3.1 note how many variables over which you now have control and are actively managing. These techniques will put those variables more strongly under your conscious control. This process will continue to bring you to higher levels of expertise and control with each exercise.

8.1 Beginner Methods

8.1.1 Modify Your Current Style with One New Concept

Don't use the template for this method; choose any single component from chapters 2 through 6 to apply within your current practice. In this case you are only using this text as a reference document.

Even though this is considered the easiest technique it can still add a fair amount of dimensionality to your teaching style.

8.1.2 Modify Your Current Style with One New Concept and a New Opening and Closing Dialogue

Don't use the template for this method; choose any single component from chapters 2 through 6 to apply within your current practice.

Also, create a new and different opening (box "e") and closing dialogue (box "p"). See chapter 1 to help with this part.

8.1.3 Modify Your Current Style with One Concept, Opening and Closing, Recurrent Themes and Class Preparation

This time use the template and choose any single component from chapters 2 through 6 and write that anywhere in section "n." Apply this technique within your current practice. Also, create a new and different opening (box "e") and closing dialogue (box "p"). Then, create some new recurrent themes (box "f") and better define your class preparation (box "d"). Write some brief notes for your new opening, closing, and recurrent themes and class preparation in the appropriate section of the template. Chapter 1 has some guidelines for these sections.

8.2 Intermediate Methods

If you wish to make the exercises in section 8.2 more challenging, use a different general series of poses for each exercise.

8.2.1 Sketching in Postures

See chapter 3 definition 3p, General Series of Poses

Design a <u>general series of poses</u> and sketch (or give the names of) those poses in the design template in section "o." Then fill in box "a" describing the general purpose for that flow.

(Tip: Use this method to capture smaller flows each in a separate template. Mix and match these flows to create new classes.)

8.2.2 Sketching in Postures and Including General Information

See chapter 3 definition 3p, General Series of Poses

Fill in the boxes from "a"-"f," then section "o" with any <u>general series of poses</u>. Do not use section "g" or curves "h," "i" and "j."

8.2.3 Sketching in Postures Including General Information and Effort Curve

See chapter 3 definition 3p, General Series of Poses and chapter 4.10

Fill in the boxes from "a"-"f," then effort level curve "h" and section "o" with a <u>general series of poses</u>. Do not use section "g" or curves "i" and "j".

Make sure that the postures properly relate to the effort curve. Remember the way the curve relates to the postures is not an exact science.

8.2.4 Sketching in Postures Including General Information and Stretch Curve

See chapter 3 definition 3p, General Series of Poses and chapter 4.10

Fill in the boxes from "a"-"f," then the stretch level curve "i" and section "o" with a <u>general series of poses</u>. Do not use section "g" or curves "h" and "j".Make sure that the postures approximately relate to the stretch curve.

8.2.5 Sketching in Postures Including General Information and Speed Curve

See chapter 3 definition 3p, General Series of Poses and chapter 4.10

Fill in the boxes from "a"-"f," then curve "j" and section "o" with a <u>general series of poses</u>. Do not use section "g" or curves "h" and "i".

Make sure that the postures approximately relate to the speed curve.

8.2.6 Sketching in Postures Including Combinations of Effort, Stretch and Speed Profiles

See chapter 3 definition 3p, General Series of Poses and chapter 4.10 and 4.11

Sketch in combinations of curves that relate to a general series of postures that you enter into section "o". In each sub-exercise, make sure that there is an approximate relationship between the curves and the postures.

Sub Exercise 1) sketch in an effort curve "h" and a stretch curve "i" against a general series of poses in section "o".
Sub Exercise 2) sketch in an effort curve "h" and a speed curve "j" against a general series of poses in section "o".
Sub Exercise 3) sketch in an stretch curve "i" and a speed curve "j" against a general series of poses in section "o".
Sub Exercise 4) sketch in an effort curve "h," a stretch curve "i" and a speed curve "j" against a general series of poses in section "o".

8.2.7 Sketching in Postures Including General Information and Pose Progression

See chapter 3 definition 3p, General Series of Poses

Fill in the boxes from "a"-"f," then column "g" and section "o" with a <u>general series of poses</u>. Do not use curves "h," "i," or "j". For example choose a set of pose categories (definition 3k) like sitting, standing, inversions, backbends, and so on. Then arrange those categories in a specific order to form your progression (definition 3l). Write your categories in this specific order into the boxes of column "g". Note that you might have a lot of poses in some categories that may require that you enter that category name into more than one box so that it as closely as possible relates to those postures in the rows of section "o".

Make sure that the pose progression you have defined in column "g" approximately relates to the postures in section "o".

8.2.8 Sketching in Postures including General information, Pose Progression and all Curves

Now let's put it all together!

See chapter 3 definition 3p, General Series of Poses

Fill in the boxes from "a"-"f," then column "g," also include curves "h," "i" and "j". Then fill in section "o" with a <u>general series of poses</u>. Make sure that the postures approximately relate to the pose progression in column "g" and curves "h," "i" and "j".

8.3 Advanced Intermediate Methods

8.3.1 General Series Method

When designing a class with a specific subject, also consider the fitness level of your students.

Chapter 3 definition 3p defines a General Series

Step 1 Fill in sections "a" through "f".
Step 2 Sketch in curves "h," "i" and "j" in such a way that it both supports the subject matter and the fitness level of your class.

Step 3 In section "g," lay out of the rough progression of your class. You may wish to start with some standing postures then move to table, inversions, postures on the back, and so on. This progression should relate to the type of class you are trying to design and also the curves "h," "i" and "j".

Step 4 Considering the posture type in section "g" and the approximate levels of effort, stretch, and speed defined in curves "h," "i" and "j," lay out a <u>general series</u> of poses that suit those requirements in section "o". The requirements set up in sections "g," "h," "i" and "j" are only a rough guide-line to help you design your class. We will never meet these requirements exactly; some ideas will blend over into other rows as you continue to fill in the postures for your class.

Up to step 4 this method is the same as 8.2.7. Now we will add steps 5 through 9. Step 5 below refers to modifications that you would make to a pose once you have established it. You may change its effort; you may animate it; you may extend limbs; you may work more on balancing; and so on. At this point go back and review chapter 4 for ideas on modifying the core poses. You can put notes for posture modification concepts in the boxes of section "o" or sec-tion "n".

Step 5 Fill in section "n" with any special notes; also include posture modification concepts from Chapter 4.
Step 6 Refer to chapter 2 for core aspects of the breath. Review against your breath ideas for possible modifications.
Step 7 Refer to chapter 5 for concepts on the edge. Apply these where necessary.

Step 8 Refer to chapter 6 for issues concerning special-needs students.

Step 9 Fill in section "p" with any notes you would like to include on shavasana.

8.3.2 Copied Series Method

Chapter 3 definition 3q defines an Imitated or Copied Series.

Since in this method we are starting with a very specific pre-determined set of poses, we will begin with those poses and then fill in the other sections of the template to suit.

Step 1 Lay out an <u>imitated or (copied) series </u>of poses in section "o" by simply sketching them into the boxes. Put the first pose into box 1, the second pose into box 2, and so on. If you have more than 48 poses you may wish to put more than one pose per box. You may have several poses of a similar type or ones that have a right to left or front to back expression; you may consider putting those into just one box.

Step 2 Fill in sections "a" through "f" the best that you can.

Step 3 Sketch in curves "h," "i" and "j" in such a way that they support the postures in the adjacent rows. Here we are doing things in the reverse order: we put the postures in first and now we are defining how we want them executed. Remember, the important thing is that the curves approximately relate to the postures.

The requirements set up in sections "h," "i" and "j" are only a rough guideline to help you design your class. We will never meet these requirements exactly; some ideas will blend over into other rows as you continue to sketch in these curves. Don't let that bother you; it is all acceptable. Do not use section "g" for this exercise.

Step 5 Fill in section "n" with any special notes; also include posture modification concepts from Chapter 4.

Step 6 Refer to chapter 2 for core aspects of the breath. Review against your breath ideas for possible modifications.

Step 7 Refer to chapter 5 for concepts on the edge. Apply these where necessary.

Step 8 Refer to chapter 6 for issues concerning special-need students.

Step 9 Fill in section "p" with any notes you would like to include on shavasana.

8.4 Advanced Methods

8.4.1 Major Pose Classical Expansion Method

See chapter 3, definitions 3c Major Pose, 3e Introductory Pose, 3f Counter Pose, 3g Transitional Pose

This method is probably one of the more fundamental academic techniques described in chapter 8. It will push you to study in detail the relationships between major, introductory, counter, and transitional poses. Here we are seeking to define a whole class using this technique. We will be choosing a set of major poses to suit a specific class subject and then we will blend them together with introductory, counter, and transitional poses.

Step 1 Fill in sections "a" through "f".

Step 2 Sketch in curves "h," "i" and "j" in such a way that it both supports the subject matter and the fitness level of your class.

Step 3 In section "g," lay out the rough progression of your class. For example, you may wish to start with some standing postures then move to table, inversions, postures on your back, and so on.

There are four columns in section "o" for a reason.

Consider that the:

1st column of boxes	1, 5, 9, 13, 17, 21, 25, 29, 33, 37, 41 and 45 are only for introductory poses.
2nd column of boxes	2, 6, 10, 14, 18, 22, 26, 30, 34, 38, 42 and 46 are only for major poses.
3rd column	3, 7, 11, 15, 19, 23, 27, 31, 35, 39, 43 and 47 are only for counter poses.
4th column of boxes	4, 8, 12, 16, 20, 24, 28, 32, 36, 40, 44 and 48 are only for transitional poses.

If you happen to choose a pose that has a right- and left-hand expression or a front to back expression simply make one side the major pose and the other side the counter pose.

Step 4 Considering the posture type in section "g" and the approximate levels of effort, stretch, and speed defined in curves "h," "i" and "j," lay out a series of <u>major poses (definition 3c)</u> that suit those requirements in the second column (start with box 2). Then continue by sketching in a series of introductory poses (definition 3e) in column 1 (start with box 1). For example the introductory pose in box 1 is an introductory pose for the major pose in box 2. In the third column (start with box 3), lay out a series of counter poses (definition 3f). For example, the counter pose in box 3 would counter the major pose in box 2. Finally in column four (starting with box 4) include a series of transitional poses (definition 3g). The transitional pose in box 4 attempts to make a smooth transition between the counter pose in box 3 and the next introductory pose in box 5.

The relationships defined above would then pertain to all of the boxes in section "o".

Again this is not an exact science; do the best you can.

Step 5 Fill in section "n" with any special notes; also include posture modification concepts from Chapter 4.

Step 6 Refer to chapter 2 for core aspects of the breath. Review against your breath ideas for possible modifications.

Step 7 Refer to chapter 5 for concepts on the edge. Apply these where necessary.

Step 8 Refer to chapter 6 for issues concerning special-needs students.

Step 9 Fill in section "p" with any notes you would like to include on shavasana.

8.4.2 Creating a Smooth Flow Series

See chapter 3 definition 3o Smooth Series

A smooth flow series, in general, is not bound by the major pose expansion techniques described above. A smooth flow series primarily seeks to be as fluid as possible.

Step 1 Fill in sections "a" through "f".

Step 2 Sketch in curves "h," "i" and "j" in such a way that it both supports the subject matter and the fitness level of your class.

Step 3 In section "g," lay out of the rough progression of your class. For example, you may wish to start with some standing postures then move to table, inversions, postures on the back, and so on.

Step 4 Considering the posture type in section "g" and the approximate levels of effort, stretch, and speed defined in curves "h," "i" and "j" , lay out a smooth series of poses in section "o". Each pose should blend extremely well to the next throughout the whole series of postures. There are some inherent health benefits to such a sequence because it will tend to not activate some of the protective reflexes in the body. Activating reflexes tends to create tension.

Step 5 Fill in section "n" with any special notes; also include posture modification concepts from Chapter 4.

Step 6 Refer to chapter 2 for core aspects of the breath. Review against your breath ideas for possible modifications.

Step 7 Refer to chapter 5 for concepts on the edge. Apply these where necessary.

Step 8 Refer to chapter 6 for issues concerning special-needs students.

Step 9 Fill in section "p" with any notes you would like to include on shavasana.

8.4.3 Creating a Strengthening Stretching Series

See chapter 3 definition 3h, Strengthening Stretching Series

Step 1 Fill in sections "a" through "f".
Step 2 Sketch in curves "h," "i" and "j" in such a way that it both supports the subject matter and the fitness level of your class.
Step 3 In section "g," lay out the rough progression of your class. For example, you may wish to start with some standing postures then move to table, inversions, postures on the back and so on.

Step 4 Considering the posture type in section "g" and the approximate levels of effort, stretch, and speed defined in curves "h," "i" and "j," lay out a <u>strengthening stretching series</u> of poses in section "o". A strengthening stretching series alternates between strengthening and stretching poses for the same muscle group. Then you would move to the next muscle group.

Step 5 Fill in section "n" with any special notes; also include posture modification concepts from Chapter 4.
Step 6 Refer to chapter 2 for core aspects of the breath. Review against your breath ideas for possible modifications.
Step 7 Refer to chapter 5 for concepts on the edge. Apply these where necessary.
Step 8 Refer to chapter 6 for issues concerning special-needs students.

Step 9 Fill in section "p" with any notes you would like to include on shavasana.

8.4.4 Creating a Multiple Stretching Strengthening Series

See chapter 3 definition 3i, Multiple Strengthening Stretching Series

Step 1 Fill in sections "a" through "f".
Step 2 Sketch in curves "h," "i" and "j" in such a way that it both supports the subject matter and the fitness level of your class.
Step 3 In section "g," lay out of the rough progression of your class. For example, you may wish to start with some standing postures then move to table, inversions, postures on the back, and so on.

Step 4 Considering the posture type in section "g" and the approximate levels of effort, stretch, and speed defined in curves "h," "i" and "j," lay out a <u>multiple strengthening stretching series</u> of poses in section "o". A multiple strengthening stretching series lays out a series of strengthening postures and then a series of and stretching postures for the same muscle group. Then you would move to the next muscle group.

Step 5 Fill in section "n" with any special notes; also include posture modification concepts from Chapter 4.
Step 6 Refer to chapter 2 for core aspects of the breath. Review against your breath ideas for possible modifications.
Step 7 Refer to chapter 5 for concepts on the edge. Apply these where necessary.

Step 8 Refer to chapter 6 for issues concerning special-needs students.

Step 9 Fill in section "p" with any notes you would like to include on shavasana.

8.5 Expert Methods

8.5.1 Creating a Contiguous Series

See chapter 3 definition 3n, Contiguous Series of Poses

Step 1 Fill in sections "a" through "f".

Step 2 Sketch in curves "h," "i" and "j" in such a way that it both supports the subject matter and the fitness level of your class.

Step 3 In section "g," lay out of the rough progression of your class. For example, you may wish to start with some seated postures then move to table, kneeling, standing, postures on the back, and so on.

Step 4 Considering the posture type in section g and the approximate levels of effort, stretch, and speed defined in curves "h," "i" and "j," lay out a contiguous series of poses in section "o". A contiguous series of poses begins in one area of the body and progresses step by step to another. For example, you may begin with poses for the feet then progress to the calves, the thighs, hips, abdomen, the chest, the neck, and finally the head. You could also start with the abdomen and move to the legs. Then back to the abdomen and move to the arms and head.

Step 5 Fill in section "n" with any special notes; also include posture modification concepts from Chapter 4.

Step 6 Refer to chapter 2 for core aspects of the breath. Review against your breath ideas for possible modifications.

Step 7 Refer to chapter 5 for concepts on the edge. Apply these where necessary.

Step 8 Refer to chapter 6 for issues concerning special-needs students.

Step 9 Fill in section "p" with any notes you would like to include on shavasana.

8.5.2 Creating an Intentional Series

See chapter 3 definition 3m, Intentional Series of Poses

Step 1 Fill in sections "a" through "f".

Step 2 Sketch in curves "h," "i" and "j" in such a way that it both supports the subject matter and the fitness level of your class.

Step 3 In section "g," lay out of the rough progression of your class. For example, you may wish to start with some standing postures then move to table, inversions, postures on the back, and so on.

Step 4 Considering the posture type in section g and the approximate levels of effort, stretch, and speed defined in curves "h," "i" and "j," lay out an intentional series of poses in section "o". An intentional series of poses is one that has a very logical connection between the major poses in terms of health benefits to the body. For example if your class subject were for the back and spine you might proceed like this: Begin with a set of postures that warm up the back in all six degrees of movement. You might then proceed with a set of postures that stretch the easier degree of movements first like front to back. Then you could proceed to the next most difficult side to side. Lastly you could stretch with the more difficult twisting postures. See how there is an added functional relationship between the postures.

Step 5 Fill in section "n" with any special notes; also include posture modification concepts from Chapter 4.

Step 6 Refer to chapter 2 for core aspects of the breath. Review against your breath ideas for possible modifications.

Step 7 Refer to chapter 5 for concepts on the edge. Apply these where necessary.

Step 8 Refer to chapter 6 for issues concerning special-need students.

Step 9 Fill in section "p" with any notes you would like to include on shavasana.

8.5.3 Creating a Free Associated Series

See chapter 3 definition, 3r Free Associated Series

Step 1 Fill in sections "a" through "f".

Step 2 Sketch in curves "h," "i" and "j" in such a way that it both supports the subject matter and the fitness level of your class.

Step 3 In section "g," do not put anything.

Step 4 In this step do not fill in any information in section "o". You will <u>free associate a series </u>of postures when you teach the class. To do this, study all of the information you have put into the template and use only that to make up your postures on the spot (or free associate). If you like you can put some general comments on posture types into section "o" and "g". But these should just be rough notes.

Step 5 Fill in section "n" with any special notes; also include posture modification concepts from Chapter 4.
Step 6 Refer to chapter 2 for core aspects of the breath. Review against your breath ideas for possible modifications.
Step 7 Refer to chapter 5 for concepts on the edge. Apply these where necessary.
Step 8 Refer to chapter 6 for issues concerning special-needs students.
Step 9 Fill in section "p" with any notes you would like to include on shavasana.

8.5.4 Creating a Combined Series

See chapter 3 definition 3s, Combined Series

Step 1 Fill in sections "a" through "f".
Step 2 Sketch in curves "h," "i" and "j" in such a way that it both supports the subject matter and the fitness level of your class.
Step 3 In section "g," lay out of the rough progression of your class. For example, you may wish to start with some standing postures then move to table, inversions, postures on the back, and so on.

Step 4 Considering the posture type in section g and the approximate levels of effort, stretch, and speed defined in curves "h," "i" and "j," lay out a <u>combined series </u>of poses in section "o". A combined series of poses employees any combination of the definitions in chapter 3 from 3d through

3u. Mix and match these techniques to come up with some highly innovative classes. Using this technique you'll see some pretty creative classes. Let your creativity soar to come up with some very novel approaches to yoga class design.

Step 5 Fill in section "n" with any special notes; also include posture modification concepts from Chapter 4.

Step 6 Refer to chapter 2 for core aspects of the breath. Review against your breath ideas for possible modifications.

Step 7 Refer to chapter 5 for concepts on the edge. Apply these where necessary.

Step 8 Refer to chapter 6 for issues concerning special-needs students.

Step 9 Fill in section "p" with any notes you would like to include on shavasana.

8.6 Advanced Expert

8.6.1 Creating a Free Associated / Intentional / Smooth Flow Series

See chapter 3 definition 3r, Free Associated Series
See chapter 3 definition 3m, Intentional Series of Poses
See chapter 3 definition 3o, Smooth Flow Series

Step 1 Fill in sections "a" through "f".

Step 2 Sketch in curves "h," "i" and "j" in such a way that it both supports the subject matter and the fitness level of your class.

Step 3 In section "g," put nothing.

Step 4 In this step do not fill in any information in section "o". You will attempt to <u>free associate</u> a series of postures that are an <u>intentional series</u> and have a <u>smooth flow</u> when you teach the class. To do this study all of the information you have put into the template and use only that to make up your postures on the spot (or free associate).

Step 5 Fill in section "n" with any special notes; also include posture modification concepts from Chapter 4.
Step 6 Refer to chapter 2 for core aspects of the breath. Review against your breath ideas for possible modifications.
Step 7 Refer to chapter 5 for concepts on the edge. Apply these where necessary.
Step 8 Refer to chapter 6 for issues concerning special-needs students.
Step 9 Fill in section "p" with any notes you would like to include on shavasana.

8.6.2 Creating a Free Associated / Contiguous / Smooth Flow Series

See chapter 3 definition 3r, Free Associated Series
See chapter 3 definition 3n, Contiguous Series of Poses
See chapter 3 definition 3o ,Smooth Flow Series

Step 1 Fill in sections "a" through "f".
Step 2 Sketch in curves "h," "i" and "j" in such a way that it both supports the subject matter and the fitness level of your class.
Step 3 In section "g," put nothing.

Step 4 In this step do not fill in any information in section "o". You will attempt to <u>free associate</u> a series of postures that are contiguous and have a smooth flow when you teach the class. To do this study all of the information you have put into the template and use only that to make up your postures on the spot (or free associate).

Step 5 Fill in section "n" with any special notes; also include posture modification concepts from Chapter 4.

Step 6 Refer to chapter 2 for core aspects of the breath. Review against your breath ideas for possible modifications.

Step 7 Refer to chapter 5 for concepts on the edge. Apply these where necessary.

Step 8 Refer to chapter 6 for issues concerning special-need students.

Step 9 Fill in section "p" with any notes you would like to include on shavasana.

8.6.3 Creating a Free Associated / Combined / Smooth Flow Series

See chapter 3 definition 3r, Free Associated Series
See chapter 3 definition 3s, Combined Series
See chapter 3 definition 3o, Smooth Flow Series

Step 1 Fill in sections "a" through "f".

Step 2 Sketch in curves "h," "i" and "j" in such a way that it both supports the subject matter and the fitness level of your class.

Step 3 In section "g," put nothing.

Step 4 In this step do not fill in any information in section "o". You will attempt to free associate a series of postures that are a combined series and have a smooth flow when you teach the class. To do this study all of the information you have put into the template and use only that to make up your postures on the spot (or free associate).

Step 5 Fill in section "n" with any special notes; also include posture modification concepts from Chapter 4.

Step 6 Refer to chapter 2 for core aspects of the breath. Review against your breath ideas for possible modifications.

Step 7 Refer to chapter 5 for concepts on the edge. Apply these where necessary.

Step 8 Refer to chapter 6 for issues concerning special-needs students.

Step 9 Fill in section "p" with any notes you would like to include on shavasana.

8.7 Closing Comments

See figure 8.1.1 for a general image on how to fill in the class design template.

At this point I would recommend going back to the introduction and reviewing sections 0.2 and 0.4 to set the framework and possibilities for application.

Whenever making changes to your teaching style, it is good to start slowly and progress gradually. Life is very complicated. If you start by making small changes, letting them stabilize and integrate into your routine, you have a much better chance for success. Then continue this process by taking on another set of small changes. Try not to go into the "New Year's Eve" syndrome where you make so many changes that it burns you out and you then discard those good changes as "just too hard".

To the contrary, I'm sure there are those people who can apply new concepts more aggressively where they become stable and permanent parts of their routine.

I have presented a lot of concepts here and a fair cross section on how to use them. Use them as is or be flexible, inventive, and creative and come up with your own new and novel ways of using this text. The possibilities are endless and can help guide your growth and development throughout your teaching career.

Enjoy!

a) Subject and Purpose: Create a general purpose class with a fair amount of effort.	b) Author: David Trimboli Date: 06 / 22 / 2008 Program : Class: of Single Class: yes	c) References: Shala Notes
d) Preparation: Room temp 70 to 75 degrees Lighting is soft Put on music CD	e) Opening Dialogue: Encourage to honor edge Let go of outside commitment Orient students to breath	f) Recurrent Themes: Keep breath full Stay aware of edge Distractions arise and pass

g) P
h) Effort —
i) Stretch - - -
j) Speed • • •

k) See definitions 3c to 3j for basic pose classifications
l) See definitions 3m to 3u for pose series concepts
m) See chapter 4 posture modification concepts

n) Notes:

Pos	o)1	2 Twist Right	3 Twist Left	4	
Sit	o)1	2 Twist Right	3 Twist Left	4	
Sit	5	6	7	8	
Table	9	10 Cat	11 Cow	12	
Lunge	13	14 Lunge Lt	15 Lunge Rt	16	
Lunge	17 Pigeon Rt	18	19 Pigeon Left	20	Animate this row, do 3x
Stand	21	22	23	24	
Back	25 Up Down	26 Up Down	27	28 Camel	Hold these poses longer
Lunge	29	30	31 Fwd Fold	32 Dog	Hold these poses longer
Invert	33 Bridge	34 Wheel	35	36	
Stand	37	38	39	40	
Stand	41	42	43	44	
Back	45	46	47 Side to Side	48 Frt to Back	

p) Shavasana / Awakening Dialogue / Closing Dialogue:
Awakening: Fingers / toe movement, rotate wrist / ankles, full body stretch, roll on right side, back to easy pose. Thank you for sharing your practice ......   Namaste'

Figure 8.1.1 Yoga Class Design Template Example (by: David Trimboli)

List of Images

List of Definitions

Index

References

[1] Zador, Veronica. Yoga Shala of Namaste Yoga, Namaste Yoga Center, Royal Oak, Mi. Sept 2000 – Jan 2001

[2] Oxford English Dictionary, Breath, Oxford University Press, on CD-ROM, Version 2.0, 2000

[3] Gray, Henry (1821–1865). "Anatomy of the Human Body." Ed. Warren H. Lewis, Philadelphia: Lea & Febiger,1918, Chapter X. The Organs of the Senses and the Common Integument, 1b. The Organ of Smell, Paragraph 14, 24, 26, Fig 855
New York: Bartleby.com, 2000 <http://www.bartleby.com/107/223.html>

[4] Gray, Henry (1821–1865). "Anatomy of the Human Body." Ed. Warren H. Lewis, Philadelphia: Lea & Febiger,1918, Chapter XI. Splanchnology, 2c. The Pharynx, Paragraph 1,2,13, Fig 1030, 1031
New York: Bartleby.com, 2000 <http://www.bartleby.com/107/244.html>

[5] Gray, Henry (1821–1865). "Anatomy of the Human Body." Ed. Warren H. Lewis, Philadelphia: Lea & Febiger,1918, Chapter XI. Splanchnology, 1a. The Larynx, Paragraph 1,3,30,35,60-66, Fig's 951, 953, 955
New York: Bartleby.com, 2000 <http://www.bartleby.com/107/236.html>

[6] Gray, Henry (1821–1865). "Anatomy of the Human Body." Ed. Warren H. Lewis, Philadelphia: Lea & Febiger,1918, Chapter XI. Splanchnology, 1b. The Trachea and Bronchi, Paragraph 1,7, Fig 961
New York: Bartleby.com, 2000 <http://www.bartleby.com/107/237.html>

[7] Gray, Henry (1821–1865). "Anatomy of the Human Body." Ed. Warren H. Lewis, Philadelphia: Lea & Febiger,1918, Chapter XI. Splanchnology, 1e. The Lungs, Paragraph 1, 21-27, Fig's 971, 974, 975
New York: Bartleby.com, 2000 <http://www.bartleby.com/107/240.html>

[8] "Alveoli." Johns Hopkins School of Medicine's, Interactive Respiratory Physiology, Copyright © 1995 Johns Hopkins University
<http://oac.med.jhmi.edu/res_phys/Encyclopedia/Alveoli/Alveoli.HTML>

[9] Matthias Ochs, Jens R. Nyengaard, Anja Jung, Lars Knudsen, Marion Voigt, Thorsten Wahlers, Joachim Richter and Hans Jørgen G. Gundersen . "The Number of Alveoli in the Human Lung," American Journal of Respiratory and

Critical Care Medicine Vol 169. pp. 120–124, (2004), © 2004 American Thoracic Society
<http://ajrccm.atsjournals.org/cgi/content/short/169/1/120>

[10] "Muscles of Respiration." Johns Hopkins School of Medicine's, Interactive Respiratory Physiology, Copyright © 1995 Johns Hopkins University
<http://oac.med.jhmi.edu/res_phys/Encyclopedia/MusclesOfResp/MusclesOfResp.HTML>

[11] Gray, Henry (1821–1865). "Anatomy of the Human Body." Ed. Warren H. Lewis, Philadelphia: Lea & Febiger,1918, Chapter IV. Myology, 6c. The Muscles of the Thorax, Paragraph 15, 30-39, Fig's 390, 391
New York: Bartleby.com, 2000 <http://www.bartleby.com/107/117.html>

[12] Coulter, David H. "Anatomy of Hatha Yoga." Body and Breath Inc., Honesdale, PA, 2001, Pg 74–76

[13] Gray, Henry (1821–1865). "Anatomy of the Human Body." Ed. Warren H. Lewis, Philadelphia: Lea & Febiger,1918, Chapter IV. Myology, 6c. The Muscles of the Thorax, Paragraph 3, 4, 6, 34, Fig 411
New York: Bartleby.com, 2000 <http://www.bartleby.com/107/117.html>

[14] Gray, Henry (1821–1865). "Anatomy of the Human Body." Ed. Warren H. Lewis, Philadelphia: Lea & Febiger,1918, Chapter IV. Myology, 5e. The Lateral Vertebral Muscles , Paragraph 2-4,7, Fig 387
New York: Bartleby.com, 2000 <http://www.bartleby.com/107/114.html>

[15] Gray, Henry (1821–1865). "Anatomy of the Human Body."
Ed. Warren H. Lewis, Philadelphia: Lea & Febiger,1918,
Chapter IV. Myology, 5b. The Lateral Cervical Muscles,
Paragraph 8, 12, Fig's 385
New York: Bartleby.com, 2000 <http://www.bartleby.
com/107/111.html>

[16] Gray, Henry (1821–1865). "Anatomy of the Human Body."
Ed. Warren H. Lewis, Philadelphia: Lea & Febiger,1918,
Chapter IV. Myology, 6d. The Muscles and Fasciae of the
Abdomen, Paragraph 6, 23, 27, 28, 36, Fig's 392, 397
New York: Bartleby.com, 2000 <http://www.bartleby.
com/107/118.html>

[17] Gray, Henry (1821–1865). "Anatomy of the Human Body."
Ed. Warren H. Lewis, Philadelphia: Lea & Febiger,1918,
Chapter XI. Splanchnology, 1c. The Pleurae, Paragraph 1,
Fig's 965, 966, 968
New York: Bartleby.com, 2000 <http://www.bartleby.
com/107/238.html>

[18] David W. Rodenbaugh, Heidi L. Collins and Stephen E. Dicarlo.
"A Simple Model for Understanding Cohesive Forces of the
Intrapleural Space." Advances in Physiological Education 27:
42-43, 2003, © 2003 American Physiological Society <http://
advan.physiology.org/cgi/content/full/27/1/42>

[19] "Alveolar Pressure." Johns Hopkins School of Medicine's,
Interactive Respiratory Physiology, Copyright © 1995 Johns
Hopkins University <http://oac.med.jhmi.edu/res_phys/
Encyclopedia/AlveolarPressure/AlveolarPressure.HTML>

[20] Edgar Lee Masters (1868–1950), "Thomas Trevelyan,"Spoon River Anthology.1916. <http://www.bartleby.com/84/151.html>

[21] Coulter, David H. "Anatomy of Hatha Yoga." Body and Breath Inc., Honesdale, PA, 2001, Pg 91–93

[22] "Dead Space." Johns Hopkins School of Medicine's, Interactive Respiratory Physiology, Copyright © 1995 Johns Hopkins University < http://oac.med.jhmi.edu/res_phys/Encyclopedia/DeadSpace/DeadSpace.HTML>

[23] Davis R. S. "Equation for the Determination of the Density of Moist Air (1981/91)." Bureau International des Poids et Mesures, F-92312, Sevres Cedex, France, Equation 1 Page 67

[24] Jones, Frank E. "The Air Density Equation and the Transfer of the Mass Unit." Institute for Basic Standards National Bureau of Standards, Washington, D.C. 20234, July 1977, Table 1, page 4 <http://ts.nist.gov/MeasurementServices/Calibrations/upload/77-1278.PDF>

[25] Wordsworth, William (1770–1850). "We are Seven." The Complete Poetical Works. London: Macmillan and Co., 1888 <http://www.bartleby.com/145/ww124.html>

[26] Thich Nhat Hanh. "Peace Is Every Step : The Path of Mindfulness in Everyday Life." Bantam Books, New York, New York, 1992 < http://thinkexist.com/quotation/smile-breathe-and-go/347521.html>

[27] Lao Tzu (approx 500 BC), "TAO TE CHING (excerpt from On the Sun and the Shade)," Translated by Raymond B. Blakney 1955 <http://www.mountainman.com.au/tao_5_9.html >

[28] Swami Vishnu-devananda. "The Complete Illustrated Book of Yoga," Three Rivers Press, New York, Pg 324–345 Copyright 1988

[29] Schiffmann, Erich. "The Spirit and Practice of Moving into Stillness," Pocket Books, New York, Pg 72–75 Copyright 1996

[30] Gray, Henry (1821–1865). "Anatomy of the Human Body." Ed. Warren H. Lewis, Philadelphia: Lea & Febiger,1918, III. Syndesmology 4. The Kind of Movement Admitted in Joints, Paragraph 3
New York: Bartleby.com, 2000 <http://www.bartleby.com/107/71.html>

[31] "Joint Articulations," Exercise Prescription on the Net, ©1999–2009 ExRx.net LLC
< http://www.exrx.net/Lists/Articulations.html >

[32] Palastanga, Nigel, Derek Field, Roger Soames. "Anatomy and Human Movement , Structure and Function." Fifth Edition, Butterworth Heinemann Elsevier, Philadelphia, Pa. Copyright 2006, Pg 4, 82, 280

[33] Oxford English Dictionary, Pronate, Oxford University Press, on CD-ROM, Version 2.0, 2000

[34] Oxford English Dictionary, Supinate, Oxford University Press, on CD-ROM, Version 2.0, 2000

[35] Palastanga, Nigel, Derek Field, Roger Soames. "Anatomy and Human Movement , Structure and Function." Fifth Edition, Butterworth Heinemann Elsevier, Philadelphia, Pa. Copyright 2006, Pg 4, 420

[36] Gray, Henry (1821–1865). "Anatomy of the Human Body." Ed. Warren H. Lewis, Philadelphia: Lea & Febiger,1918, III. Syndesmology 4. The Kind of Movement Admitted in Joints, Paragraph 5
New York: Bartleby.com, 2000 <http://www.bartleby.com/107/71.html>

[37] Palastanga, Nigel, Derek Field, Roger Soames. "Anatomy and Human Movement , Structure and Function." Fifth Edition, Butterworth Heinemann Elsevier, Philadelphia, Pa. Copyright 2006, Pg 4, 174

[38] Palastanga, Nigel, Derek Field, Roger Soames. "Anatomy and Human Movement , Structure and Function." Fifth Edition, Butterworth Heinemann Elsevier, Philadelphia, Pa. Copyright 2006, Pg 3–4, 162, 381, 348–350

[39] Gray, Henry (1821–1865). "Anatomy of the Human Body." Ed. Warren H. Lewis, Philadelphia: Lea & Febiger,1918, III. Syndesmology 4. The Kind of Movement Admitted in Joints, Paragraph 4
New York: Bartleby.com, 2000 <http://www.bartleby.com/107/71.html>

[40] Gray, Henry (1821–1865). "Anatomy of the Human Body." Ed. Warren H. Lewis, Philadelphia: Lea & Febiger,1918, III. Syndesmology 4. The Kind of Movement Admitted in Joints, Paragraph 5

New York: Bartleby.com, 2000 <http://www.bartleby. com/107/71.html>

[41] Palastanga, Nigel, Derek Field, Roger Soames. "Anatomy and Human Movement , Structure and Function." Fifth Edition, Butterworth Heinemann Elsevier, Philadelphia, Pa. Copyright 2006, Pg 4, 149, 349–350

[42] Palastanga, Nigel, Derek Field, Roger Soames. "Anatomy and Human Movement , Structure and Function." Fifth Edition, Butterworth Heinemann Elsevier, Philadelphia, Pa. Copyright 2006, Pg 64, 649

[43] Palastanga, Nigel, Derek Field, Roger Soames. "Anatomy and Human Movement , Structure and Function." Fifth Edition, Butterworth Heinemann Elsevier, Philadelphia, Pa. Copyright 2006, Pg 64, 649

[44] Gray, Henry (1821–1865). "Anatomy of the Human Body." Ed. Warren H. Lewis, Philadelphia: Lea & Febiger,1918, III. Syndesmology 7d. Talocrural Articulation or Ankle-joint, Paragraph 12
New York: Bartleby.com, 2000 <http://www.bartleby. com/107/95.html>

[45] Palastanga, Nigel, Derek Field, Roger Soames. "Anatomy and Human Movement , Structure and Function." Fifth Edition, Butterworth Heinemann Elsevier, Philadelphia, Pa. Copyright 2006, Pg 4, 411

[46] Palastanga, Nigel, Derek Field, Roger Soames. "Anatomy and Human Movement , Structure and Function." Fifth

Edition, Butterworth Heinemann Elsevier, Philadelphia, Pa. Copyright 2006, Pg 4

[47] Priebe, Dawn. Yoga Shala of Namaste Yoga (Internship Advisor), Namaste Yoga Center, Royal Oak, Mi. Sept 2000 – Jan 2001

[48] Schiffmann, Erich. "The Spirit and Practice of Moving into Stillness," Pocket Books, New York, Pg 75–78 Copyright 1996

Made in the USA
Charleston, SC
01 April 2010